THE COLON CANCER
SURVIVORS' GUIDE

Also by Curtis Pesmen

How a Man Ages

What She Wants: A Man's Guide to Women

Your First Year of Marriage

When a Man Turns Forty

THE COLON CANCER
SURVIVORS' GUIDE
Living Stronger, Longer

Curtis Pesmen

TATRA PRESS, LLC   &   BoCo MEDIA, LLC

MORRISTOWN, NJ   BOULDER, CO

Tatra Press LLC
BoCo Media LLC

Library of Congress Control Number: 2004112975
ISBN: 978-0-9776142-6-4

Designed by: Allison Ryan, Ryan Design, Bedford, NY
Editorial research and reporting by: Viki Psihoyos
Distributed by National Book Network (NBN),
Lanham, MD (800) 462-6420
Printed and bound in the United States of America by
Quebecor World Printing

Publisher contact: Chris Sulavik, Tatra Press LLC,
tatrapress@hotmail.com

Publishers' Note: This book is in no way intended to substitute for doctors' care. Its publishers urge readers to contact appropriately qualified health professionals for advice on any health or lifestyle changes inspired by information herein.

10 9 8 7 6 5 4 3 2 1

For Paula, Joshua and Jesse

Forever

CONTENTS

FOREWORD

Anyone who has traveled down this road, as author Curtis Pesmen has, can tell you that the journey is more intense than any reality television program could ever portray. And none of us has chosen the journey. No one in their right mind would choose something as shatteringly personal as colorectal cancer, but maybe to some extent we can choose its outcome. It's the fight of our life to which nothing compares.

In The Colon Cancer Survivors' Guide, Pesmen shares his cancer story and recovery—along with those of others—with the raw vulnerability that countless survivors have experienced. As unique as his journey has been, it has uncanny parallels to my own: not only in time period, but in the details of the treatment vigil as well. I've heard the term "ambushed" used to describe what an unprepared man or woman feels when the doctor tells you that you have cancer. (This book goes beyond, well beyond, the ambush.)

Regardless of the type of cancer you or a family member (or friend) had or have, I'd say the Survivors' Guide is a fair description of what happens to life as you know it from the first unscripted moments. This book gives the reader a window into a world that may best be described as a "new normal." It's the adjustment one must make after surgeries, chemo and radiation begins to creep into your daily vocabulary. And later, when you're in the throes of the biochemical violations that the body must endure to be "cured," sometimes it helps to scream, to talk, to ask questions, to cry. Or maybe journal your thoughts, as Pesmen does so eloquently in the pages that follow.

I'm hoping that those who read this will be touched—so they will understand that colorectal cancer has no respect for gender, age, or race. I applaud the author for sharing with others how life-changing, how devastating, colorectal cancer was for him. Praying that we'll come out of this challenge, but knowing nothing is certain, we learn many lessons from this powerful experience. Pesmen's heart, readers will find, is surely in the right place. We thank him for sharing his stories with us.

We know that the doctors can declare you cancer free, but the journey continues.

Louise Bates
Chairwoman, Colorectal Cancer Network

www.colorectal-cancer.net

— Author's Note —

A few years ago, over six months' time, a first-person account of a life-threatening colon cancer case appeared in the pages of *Esquire* magazine. The now public/private colon cancer case happened to be mine. The series appears in full in Chapter 1; excerpts also re-appear, in shaded blocks as "re-runs" on occasion throughout the text, for narrative flow. In addition, names of certain survivors and related details have been changed for privacy reasons.

My Cancer Story

(MONTH ONE)

MAD COLON DISEASE

At first, I thought it was the lousy British food. I had landed in London in mid-June and succumbed to a wicked case of jet jag. Or so I thought. A week, two, then three went by, and still I wasn't sleeping through the night. Restless; not in any pain, just not sleeping, and I hadn't been eating all that well, either. "Bangers and mash, buddy?" Not hardly.... My wife, Paula, and I had arrived in the UK last summer, set to stay for the better part of a year. She would serve as associate producer on the *Harry Potter* film; I'd write from overseas, traveling back and forth to the States when necessary for work....After a month or so, my sleep still somewhat restless, I notice I've lost some weight. Chris Columbus, the director [*Home Alone*, *Stepmom*] and longtime friend of mine and my wife, asks Paula one day at dinner

> " I'm scared I'm furious, I'm forty-three, and I'm fighting for my life. It's an ugly story. Here it is. "

if I'm okay; he sees I've lost weight, too. I also start to feel occasional cramps in my stomach, or lower, even, down toward my groin. Upwards of my perineum, maybe, somewhere deep down there...I also have diarrhea at least a couple of times a week (British toilet paper sucks, by the way— c'mon, the war's been over fifty-five years), which I attribute to not only the plebian British food but to the pints of warm ale that I'm trying to get used to, nightly, at the local Haverstock Arms pub.

No health ignoramus, I decide to call a doctor in London to see if what I have is a flare-up of colitis, the disease I was diagnosed with—and treated for—back in New York in 1982. I find a doc fairly easily at the Wellington Hospital, which in the two-tiered health-care system in England seems to me to treat the moneyed tier...(tea and biscuits in the lobby while we wait).

Dr. Wong takes my history and nods his head at the suggestion of colitis. Then he ushers me into the room next door. Quite polite, he asks if he can "perform" a digital rectal exam. (I assume he means on my rectum.) I say fine. And so he does, quickly. And as he removes his gloved finger, we both notice traces of blood. He asks (again politely) if he thinks we should do a flexible sigmoidoscopy—scope my large intestine—and I think not. I'll get that done back in the States, I say. And I'll be home for a week next month.... I get a prescription for some hydrocortisone foam (in other words, an uninviting suppository), which, he says, should help in the meantime....(He doesn't ask, politely, to insert the first dose.)

Looking back, I can say that both Dr. Wong and I get home that night thinking I have a case of colitis. Turns out we were wrong. We've all heard of mad cow disease—mad colon disease, maybe?

THE DIAGNOSIS [Part I]

INTERIOR: *Master bedroom of our Boulder, Colorado, home, focus on phone on nightstand next to bed.*

EXTERIOR: *Wickedly bright sunshine, some clouds over the Flatirons and foothills.*

CUE SOUND: *Phone rings.*

"Hello."

"Mr. Pesmen?"

"Yes..."

This is my doctor, my gastroenterologist, I can tell, on the line.

"Mr. Pesmen..." (Uh-oh, he's said my name twice in five seconds; not a good sign when you've been waiting for five hours for a phone call from someone who has been waiting for results from the pathology lab....)

"I've got some bad news..."

SYNOPSIS: *This is no screenplay; this is not the theater. This is (my) real life. It has just been threatened....*

SKATING AWAY [Part I]

For some reason, after I hang up with the doctor, I decide to go ahead and go ice-skating, just like I'd planned, with my friend Tom and his daughter in downtown Boulder. Call it denial, shock, incomprehension. For now, I still feel strong, I don't want to call or talk to anyone.... Paula isn't home...maybe being on the ice will somehow soothe me. I am lost, but

3

head downtown with my skates in my hands. I park the car, lock up, and hear tinny speakers blaring "Jingle Bells." Three days till Christmas....

THE DIAGNOSIS [Part II]
SCENE: *Master bedroom, still.*

"It turns out they found some cancer cells in there," the doctor says of the pathologist." I am really sorry."

I am stunned but do not cry. Instead, my body convulses slightly. Sitting on my bed, hunched over the phone, I feel as if I've just been in a minor car wreck...but all's...almost...okay. My journalistic instincts take over and I start taking notes furiously..."adenocarcinoma...second opinion...final pathology report after the weekend...need to get you to a good surgeon...don't know the stage yet...after surgery you'll know more...really sorry to give you this news...."

Merry Christmas.

SYNOPSIS: *Forget the car wreck. Feels like I have been hit by a train and have entered another world. I am now a cancer patient. December 22, 2000.*

SKATING AWAY [Part II]: MY SECRET
For an hour and fifteen minutes, I don't tell a soul. I skate and make small talk, waiting for 4:00 to arrive, when I'm supposed to pick up Paula at a friend's. She knows we've been waiting for the call and, as soon as she hops in the car, asks me if I've heard anything. I lie and say no. My secret for ten more minutes. I don't want to tell her until we get home. I feel like an ass lying to my wife about something so important, but I tell myself I'm doing it for her comfort.

When I tell her, we're in the kitchen, seated at the kitchen table.

"Paula," I say, "the doctor did call." Pause. She looks at me as if she is extremely hungry, though I know it is a look of fear.

"What? What?"

"I have cancer," I say. And nothing more.

She starts breathing heavily, then starts to shake. She starts to cry, I don't yet, then can't help but join her. Then she says she has to get down on the floor, right here, right now, or else she may faint.

My wife is now flat on her back on our white-tiled kitchen floor; we are both crying-heaving-crying, and I cradle her head in my hands and tell her to keep breathing.

"It's going to be okay," I say, not knowing if it will.

My wife and I both are now on the kitchen floor, letting this news sink in.

THE DIAGNOSIS [Part III]

SCENE: *Downtown Denver, four-story medical building.*

INTERIOR: *Surgeon's office.*

"You have rectal cancer, a kind of colon cancer," Doctor Second Opinion says. A weird dude to my eyes, kind of jumpy and unsettled, this over-eager surgeon has a good reputation among his peers. Plus he's one of the few docs we were able to see over the holidays.... Weird Dude Doc, after doing a rectal exam, then sits me in another room and compares my tumor to a rather large, gnarly bonsai tree that's thriving in a pot on his windowsill. He starts talking about growth, and I'm not liking this analogy at all. "This man will not operate on me," I think as I take copious notes, realizing that surgeons' skill has little to do with their personalities.

CUT TO: *The University of Colorado Health Sciences Center.*

INTERIOR: *Exam room of Dr. Third Opinion, Robert McIntyre, M.D.*

"I agree you have rectal cancer," Dr. McIntyre of the University of Colorado says. "The question is how much of the colon will we have to remove...." I like this guy, his manner, his calm demeanor, his apparent mastery of the diagnosis with only limited information, which is why he's prepping me for a series of CT scans later this day, ordered by Dr. Cory Sperry, a friend of ours and a friend of his, to see if any cancer has spread to my lungs, abdomen, or liver.... This guy could operate on me, I think. And after he calls two days later to tell us the CT scans look "good...I see the tumor, but the lungs, abdomen, and liver look clear," Paula and I feel like we've been given a reprieve. Good doc. Good results following a horrifying few days, and aftershock. Now, maybe, we can set up a plan to kick this cancer's ass, to turn perhaps the wrong phrase....

SYNOPSIS: *I try to focus on some of Doc McIntyre's last words to Paula and me as we huddled in the exam room: "Cancer is a word, not a sentence." I'm curable.*

TOUGH CALL

Waiting. And wondering why I'm sitting on my bed on Saturday morning, delaying the inevitable. Waiting to call my family in Chicago and tell them the news. Making the wrong call and the right call at the same time, deciding to start by calling my sister, Beth. After all, she's my only sibling, just a couple of years older, forty-five, and has been through a major assault, having lost her first husband, Art, to leukemia when he was thirty-five and she was thirty-two, a rock then; I expect her to be a rock now.

"I have cancer," I blurt after we chat about who-in-the-hell-remembers for about a minute. A slight pause. Longer pause, then a mournful wail and sob and heaving of breath and sound and emotion I have never heard emanate from my sister. Or from anyone close to me. Positively frightening. I'm now shaking, taking this in, realizing that maybe I've touched a dormant nerve that reached right back to that day when she became a widow, in July 1988.

Haunting, her sobs. "No! *Nooooooooooo, noooo!*" And then she recovers. And then we settle into the shaken rhythms of our breathing, somehow feeling stronger, if only for a minute. I grab Paula's hand a little tighter while we buck up and prepare for The Next Call.

At sixty-nine and seventy-two, my mom and dad, Sandy and Hal, are to me a model couple. Semiretired, semihip (my mom can still get away with leather pants; my dad, a leather bomber jacket), semi-serious about fitness, and married happily for nearly all of their forty-nine years together. I've got to "protect" them but can't delay any longer.

"I'm okay," I tell my mother as she asks, rhetorically, how I am. A signal from son to mother. She knows "okay" means something's wrong, though she turns out to be a rock. "I have cancer," I choke out to her, wondering if the fact that her mom died of cancer at forty-one, when she was only nine, has somehow steeled her against some of the worst medical news she could hear. My dad is a different story. He takes in the diagnosis, breaks up, then says, "You...have my colon." He repeats it. I'm confused, as my father has never had intestinal problems. He hands the phone off to my mom, shaken, and she tells me we will get through this and come out the other side....

Weeks later, I learn what my father was trying to tell me through emotional upheaval: "You can *have* my colon." At a literal loss for words, he was telling me he was willing to donate his, or part of his, large intestine to me, no matter how unlikely a scenario this could ever be. I'm glad I didn't know what he meant at the time.

NOT HOME ALONE

After Paula e-mails Chris Columbus and a few other people she's working with on the Potter movie, Chris calls our home immediately. He has put in calls to friends, including Robin and Marsha Williams, in San Francisco, to try to help us get fourth or fifth opinions at University of California, San Francisco, a top cancer center and the one that the Columbuses and Williamses have the utmost trust in…. It's also the hospital where Paula has some strong contacts, from years of helping coordinate movie screenings and benefits that have aided UCSF fundraising.

Almost unbelievably, Chris and his wife, Monica Devereux, immediately offer us the use of their home in San Francisco if we should choose to go there for treatment. And within hours, Marsha Williams is on the phone with Paula…then me…talking about how important it is to get the best doctors for cancer treatment…and that she knows how to help us find them at UCSF. An unlikely Hollywood connection to my cancer, I am thinking, but there is friendship at the core of these gestures, not glamour or glitz. I am amazed at the outreach that's seemingly coming into our world, one call at a time….

HAPPY FRICKIN' BIRTHDAY

Lashing out at Doctor Worthless in our darkened bedroom back in Boulder. We're home, "relaxing" and packing, getting used to powerful pain meds (and stool softeners to counteract their constipatory effects), and I'm still angry, I realize through late-night sobbing, at the Denver doctor who shall remain nameless, for now, who calls himself a gastroen-terologist but did not, four to five months ago (*after* Dr. Wong's bloody finger and recommendation of a sigmoidoscopy), perform even a digital rectal exam that should have discovered this two-inch-long "locally inva-sive" tumor. Laziness? Maybe. HMO pressures to see too many patients per hour? Doubt It. The worthless doc didn't see fit to look where he should have, when he should have, as most competent gastroenterologists would suggest. I stop crying, settle down for a long fight, and try to find grace in this situation on a day that is probably the worst birthday my wife Paula has ever endured.

I'm prone most of the day and unable to get to the store to buy a card or present for my partner, the love of my life, who cries as I present her, shortly after midnight; with a thirty-ninth-birthday card with thirty-nine hand-drawn hearts that I've fashioned from a folded business card of mine, drawing and writing in the bathroom between our two sinks. Happy frickin' birthday indeed.

FUTURE BEST-SELLER?

My best friend, Geoff, whom I've known since 1970, calls from Chicago: "I got an idea," he says. "You can do a book, call it: *Me, Cancer, and Geoff*. Instead of a book about how you and your wife got through this together, it'll be a buddy book about how I helped you kick cancer. I'll be calling you every day; people aren't expecting that." Pause. "You're sick," I say. "I know," he says. "But I gotta ask you: Does this mean I'll have to do one of those Run-Walk things with you in five years?"

THE DIAGNOSIS [Part IV]

SCENE: *Exterior, UCSF Surgery Faculty Practice building, 400 Parnassus Avenue, San-Francisco.*

INTERIOR: *Office of Dr. Mark Lane Welton, colorectal surgeon.*

"…I believe your case is not a slam dunk; but I don't think it's one of my fourteen-hour operations, either," Dr. Welton says in the first hour of our meeting. "It's probably a three-to four-hour operation."

We soon learn that the cancer was found very late.

"Your cancer is advanced," Dr. Welton tells us.

"Then why didn't they find it in my screening three years ago?"I snap.

Dr. Welton shakes his head and tells me, "I'd guess it's at least five years old."

SYNOPSIS: *He seems confident surgery will cure me, but he won't openly rip his colleagues. (Seems he believes Dr. Worthless and other private-practice gastros aren't as adept in colonoscopy as many practicing docs at university med centers, such as UCSF.) I like his style and honesty. If I have to be cut up, I want Dr. Welton to do the job.*

PROBING MY NODES

Lying on my back, waiting for doctor whomever from UCSF "paths" (pathology) to enter the room to do an FNA (fine-needle aspiration) of my inguinal lymph nodes, down by the groin and perineum, where the body normally doesn't invite needles in...poke, dig, poke, dig, poke, dig, he does. All negative—great! No cancer cells found. But he has to probe each one again, he tells me, a second time, to be "more sure."

Great, I'm thinking, and Dr. Daphne Haas-Kogan is still planning to zap my nodes anyway, with God knows how many radiative "Grey," for good measure, I later learn…. Gotta rush so the next docs can operate on me and insert a chemotherapy "port" in my chest...then Paula's gotta toss me on a United plane and fly my ass home for the weekend. Looks like we've made the choice: San Francisco for my treatment and surgery; back home to Colorado for the healing.

THE TEAM

Learning, in a hurry, that when you have cancer you don't have just one doctor. In my case my team includes:

- Alan Venook, M.D., forty-six, medical oncologist, UCSF

- Mark Lane Welton, M.D., forty-four, colorectal surgeon, UCSF

- Daphne Haas-Kogan, M.D., thirty-seven, radiation oncologist, UCSF

- Jonathan Terdiman, M.D., thirty-seven, gastroenterologist, UCSF

- Jerry Ashem, fifty-six, nurse, home chemotherapy provider, Life Care Solutions

- Nancy Rao, N.D., forty-four, naturopath and accupuncturist, Boulder, Colorado

- Paula Dupré Pesmen, thirty-nine, associate producer, wife, partner

EIGHT WORDS YOU DON'T WANT TO HEAR

It's something I won't soon forget...there I am, splayed out on a hard exam table in the radiation-therapy room, hospital PJ bottoms pulled halfway down my crotch...when a senior member of the rad/oncology team addresses a younger doctor after viewing my simulation—the precise position I will be in when radiation beams will enter my body. He uses eight words: "The penis is going to have a reaction." In other words, the penis (which would be mine) will very likely develop a sunburn of sorts, perhaps over six weeks of absorbing nearby radiation waves. Note to self: "Prepare."

TREATMENT: CHEMOTHERAPY

Surprise: In this new new age of personal electronics, it appears that my six weeks of chemotherapy will be administered by a machine, not a person.

Small enough to fit in a fanny pack, BlackBerryish in personality, the portable pump I name Abbott, built by Abbott Labs outside Chicago, will be in charge of delivering a toxic chemical, a toxic cancer-fighting chemical, 5-fluorouracil, into my bloodstream. (I could opt for weekly visits to an infusion center, where my medical oncologist has his office, but since I'm on a low-dose regimen, Abbott seems the way to go.) He's got a small screen, twenty-four buttons, lots of chirps and beeps, and a clear plastic tether tube that stretches about four and a half feet.

Once a week, a home nurse will come and change the medicine, flush my "line," take my blood pressure, draw some blood, change his gloves, don a mask, change the needle that fits in the port inside my chest, swab the whole upper-right quadrant of chest with antiseptic, then tape me down, making me water-resistant, not quite waterproof, for at least six weeks. More chemo later? I wonder.... Yes, I learn soon enough, but it probably won't be porta-pumped in.

TREATMENT: RADIATION

Beep. Beep. Beep. Beep.

Whirr. Whirr.

Bzzzzz. Bzzzzz. Bzzzzz...Silence.

Ker- CHUNK....

Welcome to the world of Radiation Oncology, Day One of the six-week treatment, as part of a protocol that's not practiced everywhere. Some docs say, till more data are in, the tumors should be taken surgically first, followed by chemo and radiation. But not the docs we have on our team. It's a sandwich kind of cancer-fighting. BEEP/WHIRR, then surgery; then chemo afterward, as necessary.

Today, in the basement of UCSF's Long Hospital, amid the city's first big storm of the year, I try to find a quiet moment as the Big Gun goes off. *Beep, Beep, Beep. Whirrr...Bzzzz....*

MY 24/7/6 ANTI-CANCER MACHINE

Wondering why some people are so afraid to use the word "cancer" when they e-mail or write notes to me sending warm thoughts....Thanking the literary lords that a ten-year-old daughter of one of my friends sent a card that said, up front: "Dear Curt, I hope you fight off your cancer.... Love, Rebecca"

How the hell can you take this sucker on ...if you can't call it by its name? It's cancer, and I'm hooked up to a porta-chemo-pump stashed in a fanny pack that's "pretreating" my tumor while I get daily blasts of radiation (weekends off), courtesy of the GE Clinac 2300 radio-therapy accelerator. I'm a 24/7/6 (six months total treatment) anti-cancer assault unit, with all this technology comin' at me, going in me, going through me and God knows where else into the walls of the underground radia-tion oncology unit named for Walter Haas, the Levi Strauss magnate, and dedicated in 1983.

Otherwise, it's January 2001, and, shoot, things are great.

EAT MORE, WEIGH LESS

Weighing in one afternoon while in treatment at 168. Wondering where the pounds went so quickly. I was 183 before I left for England last summer. My appetite is down, so is my general attitude toward eating. "Food is no longer for pleasure," Dr. Haas-Kogan ("Call me Daphne") says. "It's your job."

SEX AND MY CANCER

Haven't found lots of info on the standard patient Web sites about sex and colon cancer.... Here's what I know so far: In one month of being a colon-cancer patient, I've had sex twice, once what I would term successfully. The other time, well, that's what I know about sex and my cancer.

HAPPY ANNIVERSARY

One month after the diagnosis. My anger has dissipated toward my doofus doctor who never stuck his middle finger up my anus all fall 2000, while I complained of rectal pain—it's right there in his carefully written notes in the records I snatched, or rather requested, from his office. I mean, of course my anger has cooled....

Consider: A patient at higher-than-average risk of colon cancer comes in and complains of stomach pain, rectal pain, and diarrhea (some would call that "a change in bowel habits..."), and in your wisdom you decide not to perform a basic digital rectal exam. Cruel irony, perhaps, that the cancer you'd later find would show up in the rectum. And was, other surgeons have said, large enough to have been felt by a doctor's finger.... And if you had glanced through my records, you would have seen that you performed a screening colonoscopy on me a few years ago, and that I had some suspect tissue that turned out to be benign. No need to check back, I guess. I know how hard doctors have to work these days.

Four or five months earlier, diagnosis would only mean I'd be a lot more comfortable right now and have a better—as hard as it is to say—chance of cure, whatever that means in oncological parlance. You can have your five-year survival rates, Dr. Worthless. You've called me exactly once in a month's time to check on me, your patient that you recently diagnosed as having colon cancer. Remember me? Happy frickin' anniversary. Maybe see you in court.

"A POSSIBLY FATAL EVENT"

Guinea-pig Friday. Seven hours of waiting for a cautionary scan of my lungs and legs, all because I reported having shortness of breath this morning and my surgeon, Dr. Welton, and his resident scrunched their eyebrows like squirrels (if I'm a guinea pig, they're squirrels) and thought of the remote possibility of PE—pulmonary embolism—"a possibly fatal event."

I have a few risk factors, you see: an open line running into my veins for chemo; I have cancer; I am over forty years old; have an infection; and have been largely immobile. Better safe than dead, they think but don't say. (Reportedly, it's one of the most frequently missed diagnoses in medicine.) So there goes our Friday afternoon and evening. We wait, and wait, for a space in the CT queue...and Doc Daphne comes over from the hospital next door to try to help move things along...at 8:00 p.m. on a Friday night. Three kids she has at home, and she's with Paula and me. This is what you call care. This is what leads to Paula getting for her four Harry Potter T-shirts from her stash in London. My lungs and legs turn out to be clear.

A SOB STORY

Waking up with bad chemo/radiation nausea and diarrhea...an hour on the john to start the day...followed by thirty minutes of intense sobbing in bed, broken occasionally by heavy breathing (to relax me), the tears flow and I plead for "a break." I know part of this frustration is from yesterday's seven hours of helplessness and waiting for exams...and the possibility of "a fatal event," as if colorectal cancer isn't a possibly fatal event. I begin to view crying as part of healing. It's probably in the cancer-support books that the nurses gave me and that I've yet to read.... Fourth, you cry.

LICK ME

After too many days of chemo/poison pumping through my veins, my body sends its first signal of being pissed off at the assault—a rash, or rawness, on the back and center of my tongue, all raised and ugly, what the doctor calls "mucousitis"; what a nurse says might be thrush...we'll worry about it tomorrow. Today, I'll just add some antibiotics to my arsenal to try and hit the elusive fever that kicks up each afternoon and evening, from 99.4 to 100.5 or so, possibly related to last week's discovery of an abscess. "Possibly," say Dr. Daphne and Dr. Welton. Lotsa *possiblys* in this long-term anti-cancer contest that's still in the early stages. Even a temporary alarm set off by Abbott—signaling occlusion in the tubes that send 5-FU chemo drug into my body—doesn't trip us up for long.

An 800 number, plus a knowing pharmacist on the "home health care/Life Care Solutions" hotline, helps us get Abbott back on track with only a ten-minute interruption in cancer-kick-butt service. With *ER* playing in the background on TV, my little chemo emergency couldn't have asked for a more macabre backdrop. Blood and guts all over the Mitsubishi big-screen TV...a portable-CD-player-sized pump in my hands, sending peeling alarm signals and not responding to my attempted repair. And I can't very well call Dr. Greene.

I DON'T LIKE MONDAYS

Setting the alarm for 8:45 a.m., which to the rest of the world sounds late, I know, but for someone who is woken up every two hours to take a piss because radiation waves have riled up my bladder tissue till it's as angry as an eighty-four-year-old's who's got a mean case of prostatitis...truth is, I don't want to arise at 8:45. I could easily sleep till 10:00, since I haven't enjoyed real REM-type sleep for what seems like a week.

Waiting for nurse Jerry, all earnest and bearded and careful and responsible-like, to come visit and slip on the rubber gloves and rip a bent needle out of the port that's been surgically implanted in my chest...new week, new bag of "dope" for my main man, Abbott.... It's all good, I suppose, but I don't enjoy lying flat on my back with anti-splash pads beneath my chest and torso. (Chemo is poison, let's remember; we don't want that stuff splashing about the linens, much less our respective skins....)

Mondays mean a whole week ahead of whomping the bad cells with good X rays and 168 milliliters of 5-fluorouracil cocktail, my chemo drug of choice...so by Friday night or Saturday morning, I will almost certainly feel like shit. Which means, they tell me, Mondays should actually be "good" days, because I've had the weekend off from the radiation assault...and my body's had a chance to "recover."

Shoot, other than that, Mondays are fine specimens of the week. When you're normal, that is. When you're Cancer Boy, you're just a bit more skeptical about this fine day....

BONDING

Flipping off a friend, in a good way, a male-bonding way, as I lie on the couch, fatigued and diseased. He's flown twenty-five hundred miles to visit me, my old roommate Todd, and at one point I look over at him in the living room, our eyes meet, and I give him the finger. He understands completely. What men want. A tough way to say, "Thanks for leaving your job and family for a few days to come hang with me as I get chemo'd and radiated." A guy thing. I love the guy. He's here. I'm hurtin'. So "Flip off." Makes perfect sense, as Paula wonders, maybe, what in the hell I've just done to my friend. She understands, maybe not completely.

CAN CANCER BE EMBARRASSING?

An East Coast friend, whom I've known since 1980, calls: "So...it must be hard having cancer in a place that's embarrassing?"

I pause, weighing the absurdity of the comment, then respond.

"I guess so. But I guess I'd rather have colon cancer than brain cancer." Insensitive dude, I am as well, knowing that I disrobe every day in the bowels of UCSF's Long Hospital alongside patients who are being treated radiotherapeutically for cancer in and on their brains.

That's not so embarrassing? I wonder. And we go on to talk about, believe it or not, the New York Yankees.

SUNBURN WHERE THE SUN DON'T SHINE

"It's gonna get worse before it gets better;" says Doc Daphne as I hit the home stretch of "Intro to Radiation 101" (six-week course). Sunburnlike burns on my inner buttocks, burned and raw skin where groin meets thigh, and, yes, a scorched penis. Time to learn, from the radiation nurse, how to use and apply the wickedly priced, aloe-based ointment known as: Carrington RadiaCare Gel Hydrogel Wound Dressing. It's soothing, I soon find, as I hitch up my drawers and shuffle off after getting dressed, holding my wife's left hand in my right.

(MONTH TWO)

GETTING TO KNOW PAIN

Don't know why I'm surprised, five weeks into treatment, how much cancer hurts, but I am. The pain I've gotten to know, that renders me horizontal at least five hours a day, has started messing with my mind. I've been hurting at least four months now. Even with narcotics (and I have good ones), I hurt more profoundly, more often, than I can take. It is so deep inside, it actually radiates from my pelvis out into my legs and down to the soles of my feet. It gets to where I start naming the types of pain: stabbers, daggers, and achers. (Achers hurt the worst.)

Driven to the couch two/three times a day, I wonder what it would take to become part of California's legal medical-marijuana program. The docs at UCSF don't seem all that familiar with it, but they give time four phone numbers to try and a list of instructions. Gotta check this out further.

DOWN FOR THE COUNT

Whipping around the corner in Long Hospital's basement, late for my daily beams of radiation, scurrying into the men's changing room (does it *really* matter whether you wear hospital gowns and pajama bottoms instead of T-shirts and jeans when it's radiation we're talking about?), and getting undressed/dressed in almost record time....

Feeling light-headed as I wait for my appointed slot under The Gun, looking for an empty chair—"Do you want me to get you a chair?" my sister Beth says—and I say no, feeling macho, but also feeling more lightheaded than I know—*slam/crumple/thump*—I'm down on the tile floor in an instant—unconscious. Ten seconds, twenty, maybe thirty. When I come to, I see three sets of eyes staring down at me.... "Curt, Curt, can you hear me?" my wife, Paula, pleads. "I need a gurney and a pulse ox!" Doc Daphne shouts, *E.R.*-style. I am coming to...quickly...not knowing why I went down or what my elbow hit on the way down, 'cause it's hurting but not bleeding, and suddenly there are eight people hovering around me on my gurney as I "stabilize."

Wheeling me into the Rad Room, the radiation therapists ask me if I can stand. I say yes, not knowing if I can and yet not knowing that I had the beginnings of a seizure while on the ground. I quickly learn that radiation treatments *don't stop*...just 'cause a patient goes down.

Rolling into the ER upstairs moments later, I'm wired for an EKG to check my heart, and the battery of tests commences...blood, urine, neuro, orthostatics [blood pressure standing and sitting]. Bottom line, the docs think I've been dehydrated due to the chemo and other aspects of cancer treatment; and my red-blood-cell count is low.

The assault continues, as Doc Daphne checks in before my discharge to suggest that we do "a head MRI" sometime soon...takes a while for my brain to click in...she's checking for balance problems...or maybe a blood clot caused my fainting spell?...or else, well, maybe she's just gonna scan my head, MRI-style, to rule out that slim chance that I have cancer in my brain. The assault continues....

SHOWERDANCE

With a [chemo port] line going into my chest, with a four-inch-by-four-inch swatch of Tegaderm breathable-but-not-waterproof bandage on top of the contraption, I'm not allowed to take showers as I used to, before I became a cancer patient.

I wash my hair in the sink (using a plastic Pac Bell Park cup for the big-rinse finish) most days or do a quick, body-turn shower, wherein I leave my chemotherapy pump parked in its fanny pack just outside the shower door and wet what I can, soap what I can, then washcloth the rest, once

I've successfully rinsed, keeping my trusty chemo pump, "Abbott," dry.

WE GOT GAME

Walking across the street, trailing my nephew Clark, who's come to visit and, frankly, is hoping to play some hoop with his uncle. His *fatigued* uncle.

He dribbles, shoots, scores, so do I! He spins the red-and-black Harlem Globetrotter promotional basketball lazily, woozily, on his right middle finger. I catch the ball and show Clark how to spin it faster and how to get the ball to spin on my/his finger for ten seconds instead of five....

Shots go in; three-pointers clang off the rim; Paula shoots her first shot and somehow gets it stuck—lodged—between the rim brace and the back-board. I struggle to jog/run after rebounds...I'm huffing...but fact is...eighty days after my diagnosis, I am once again playing an outdoor game.

SEX AND MY CANCER [Part II]

Wondering, in bed, how long it will take for the barbecued, irradiated skin on my package to return to normal color and texture.... Finding that having an erection and doing something pleasurable with it hurts in such odd, frightening ways in the first weeks after radiation treatment...that it makes you think twice about having an erection and doing something pleasurable with it.

LEAVE YOUR DIGNITY AT THE DOOR

"Tough-ass Sim," is all I can say...and it's not a sorry pun. It's a day of Radiation Simulation I'll remember as one of the worst, particular to my type of colorectal cancer, to my type of presurgery treatment.

"Curt, you may have to leave your dignity at the door," says Doc Daphne as she leads me to a treatment room. Within minutes, I am bottomless, on my belly, on a hard table, with doctors and therapists around me, drawing Magic Marker targets on my ass and hips, calling out measurements that I don't understand. The rectal/anal probes that irritate tumor tissue I do understand. Quickly. I groan like a farm animal. This is what the good doctor meant by leaving my dignity at the door. Feeling like a roasted pig with an apple in its snout: "Come get me—I'm done."

Forty-five minutes later, my pelvis is now prepped to guide the beams of my last few radiation "boosts." "I'm sorry," Doc Daphne says of The Sim. "I'm really sorry."

FINDING GOD [Part I]

Realizing, on day seventy-one after diagnosis, in year forty-three of my life, that I have never prayed as regularly before.

WELL RUNS DRY

If it's emotional dehydration I'm worrying about, and I'm worrying about Paula's "well" often, I find a few answers in her journal:

Curt's been on chemo & radiation for weeks—he's doing okay, but he's sick and very tired and still has a fever every night. We're fighting to keep weight on him, literally. Each meal is a battle between me and a guy called Nausea. I am determined to win and I do, because losing means that I'm letting Curt down.

Today I had a meltdown. I was lying on the bed crying like a two-year-old late for a nap. I have to tell Curt, I'm tired of being the bad guy. I represent the things that bring him discomfort: food, medicine, trips to the hospital. I ride his butt each day to take a pain pill, go for treatment, eat, eat, eat.... I want to hold him and kiss him and nurture him well, but those things are just a part of his wellness. He lost 6 pounds last week and the doctor's concerned. I have to keep him eating. He's having very serious surgery soon and needs to be strong.

Cancer is trying to come between us. Where I used to lay my head, now lies a chemo port sewn into his chest. Nausea and fever cause him to need space. I tell Curt I want to be small so I can curl up in his arms and feel him. This disease is trying to isolate Curt from people he loves. I won't let it happen. He takes me to the chair where we curl up and he holds me like I'm his wife and everything feels good again. Today we've won.

The Facts

- Colorectal cancer is the second leading cause of cancer-related death in the U.S. (Lung cancer is the first.)
- Nearly 10 percent or 50,000 deaths deaths from cancer in the U.S. in 2007 were due to colorectal cancer.
- About 90 percent of people diagnosed with colon cancer are over age 50.

HIGH-RISK FACTORS INCLUDE:

1) Family history
2) A diet low in fiber and high in fat (mostly from animal sources)
3) Personal history of colon polyps
4) Personal history of chronic inflammatory bowel disease, Crohn's disease, or ulcerative colitis. People suffering from Crohn's disease or ulcerative colitis for more than 20 years are at more than twice the risk for colorectal cancer than the average person their age.

SYMPTOMS OF COLORECTAL CANCER MAY INCLUDE:

1) Rectal bleeding
2) Blood in the stool
3) A change in bowel habits
4) Abdominal, rectal, or liver pain
5) Feeling of fatigue, loss of weight, or decreased appetite.

Doctors recommend that all people over 50 receive some type of screening, at least an annual FOBT, or fecal occult blood test. The American College of Gastroenterology recommends that people over 50 receive a colonoscopy at least once every 10 years, as well as an FOBT and a flexible sigmoidoscopy once every five years.

Patients diagnosed with ulcerative colitis or Crohn's disease are at particularly high risk and should undergo colonoscopy at least once every two years.

NICE 'N' ANGRY

Getting a bill from Dr. Worthless in Denver for services "rendered"...wondering if/or how much I should pay the doctor who I believe fouled up my diagnosis and treatment for months last fall. Knowing part of what I believe is supported by my medical records. I'm still furious he never did digital rectal exams when I went to see him—twice—complaining of rectal pain last fall. There was—and is—a tumor where he could have felt it.

Thinking back to what Dr. Haas-Kogan told me not long ago about my disease: "Don't give up your license to be angry. No forty-three-year-old man should have to go through what you're going through."

My "license to be angry." I hadn't thought of things this way. Now I do.

A HEAD CASE

Driving across town in early afternoon to the shiny, happy, new UCSF Cancer Center, to get my chemo line unhooked, to get the needle removed from the port in my chest, to get back to living without being tethered to a pump/fanny pack that even has to sleep with me under my pillow. Progress. I'm free, in a way, six weeks before surgery, but tonight I have a date with my wife, my friend Jim, and the MRI machine.

The docs, the good folks taking care of me, who haggled over my fainting spell last week, are going to have a close look at my brain. They want the MRI to "rule out" cancer in my brain as a cause.... Ten times louder (slo-mo jackhammers), three times more uncomfortable (claustrophobia) than the CT scans I now know too well...the MRI of the matter inside my skull comes out pretty well...at least for now.

Bottom line: no cancer found in my brain, but, and there's always a *but*, there are two fuzzy spots on the film outside my skull that the docs may want to take a closer look at. When you have cancer, there are sound reasons sometimes to keep looking for more cancer. This means for me another round of tests in the future, a round of tests that Paula and I don't want to deal with right now. My docs give me a break, at least for now.

THE DIAGNOSIS [Part V]

EXTERIOR: *Master shot. Rolling clouds, west to east, across San Francisco Bay.*

INTERIOR: *Eighth-floor medical office, Moffitt Hospital, UCSF.*

Meeting with my surgeon a month and a half before surgery, getting ready to schedule The Date, finding out I'll need at least three more scans and four more meetings with doctors before I get cut. Learning that I'll be losing most if not all of my colon in less than two months. Slipping into journalistic mode, I shut off emotions and hear "colostomy," "ileostomy"...bagged for life. Or for at least a long time.

SYNOPSIS: *Major Lifestyle Change, a reasoned journalist might say, in exchange for Life.*

FINDING GOD [Part II]

Not realizing until my diagnosis, and until the news got out, how many friends and family members who never talk to me about religion regularly pray. Now they send word of including me in their nightly prayers and other prayer circles. A cousin of mine sends a miniature carving of a powerful-looking shaman...there's a guy I want to take into surgery with me.

HEADING HOME

Still reeling, and peeling, nine days after the last of the big radiation blasts ...no more chemo pumping into my veins; wondering how long it takes to clear my body completely (if indeed it does clear completely).

Knowing I now have 3.3 weeks left to "heal" and get stronger back home in Boulder before the surgery; trying not to think about that right now...don't know that I could even handle the trip/airport/assholes—plus-three hours of sitting—just yet...popping a Vicodin to stifle the pain...taking a walk in the park, heavy legs and all, in Pac Heights to try and beat the fatigue.

But I don't. Beginning to understand why I saw that hospital flyer about a clinical study looking for subjects re: cancer fatigue. Fatigue is no small matter. No small malady. The sucker doesn't know when to leave. It is a key part of the assault.

I want, among other things, the lightness in my legs back.

(MONTH THREE)

HIGH MILEAGE/LOW MILEAGE

Feeling like a low-mileage patient today...which means pretty good in cancer-doc speak. Hang around the oncology ward long enough and you'll hear hospital workers instantly, cruelly, assess new patients as "high mileage" or "low mileage." Which one's gonna take more work? Which one's got the better chance for cruising down the road, in years ahead?

Feeling like a human again...back home and healing after Round One of treatment. Walking slowly after lunch around the lake by our house, logging a total of 1.3 miles. High mileage, low mileage, whatever. It's actual miles, and I'm counting.

FRIENDS, FINANCES, FOOD

Settling back into our own home in Boulder after the two-month medical pilgrimage to San Francisco. Opening the first of the hospital bills with more zeros on the end than I can take seriously. Reconnecting with friends, who absolutely feel like family as they swarm the house in preordained small-group waves...the first posse sneaking in the day before our arrival and stocking the house with food.

Second wave cooks us a Saturday-night turkey-meatloaf-mashed-pots-and-gravy dinner; third wave brings over take-out Chinese...which is all good, all fine, all warm and fuzzy-like...except that in my case, food that = love also = pain—almost instant pain after eating—and that reminds me I still have an angry, invasive adenocarcinoma residing at the end of my digestive tract.

DEAD MAN SLEEPING

Trying not to think about surgery, cancer, recovery, chemo, and going back to UCSF in three weeks. Luxuriating, almost, with Paula's fresh soups, French-toast-with-strawberry breakfasts, late-night shakes to put the weight back on...and small groups of friends stopping by to check in, check on me, see how Paula's holding up....

Then a call comes, less than a week since we've been home. Her dog, our dog, Toto, the thirteen-year-old Maltese, died last night while asleep under the bed of Paula's mom in California, where he's been living for the past six months. No ordinary hound, Toto the Wonderdog. Can't help but weep through the late morning...what lousy timing. Then comes an unlikely knock on our door from a Boulder cop. Asks to come in, leads us to our living-room window, explaining that he is looking for clues....Seems a dead man was found a few hundred yards from our house, in the 6.2 acres deemed "open space" by the city.... Whether the man was murdered or died-in-his-sleep we do not know. Cop doesn't, either, or at least he's not saying. I'm hurting, pelvically, colonically, taking this all in, trying to be strong on my feet, telling Officer Navarro that I was up between 3:40 and 5:00 a.m., in bed, and didn't hear anything. We didn't do it, officer. Now can you leave us to ponder...two deaths...too close to home...while I, we, just try to recover in "paradise"?

SEX AND MY CANCER [Part III]

A wife (that would be mine) writes in her journal: "It's our 7th anniversary. I asked Curt if he had the seven-year itch. He said, 'only where the radiation burns are healing.' (That would be his groin, and that would be a 'no' to my question.)"

FRIENDLY FIRE

Walking toward Wonderland Lake, looking for the soccer field where my friend Tom is coaching his daughter and other seven-or-eight-year-olds. Hanging around with the parents, reminding myself that Paula and I aren't parents yet, and at thirty-nine and forty-three, time is running short....

Wondering why I can't remember whether—at week ten of my treatment—my sperm could ever recover and (safely) father a baby after all the radiation my groin, pelvis, and balls have been through. Thinking back to the day weeks ago when I banked sperm in that horrible windowless room in a San Francisco fertility clinic, just in case friendly fire of any sort would hurt our chances.

GOTTA HAVE FAITH

Taking a walk to boost my strength from radiation and chemo, still not quite 170 pounds. Trying not to think too much about the surgery in two weeks, but how much is too much? I can't help but think—and say to Paula— "Do you realize we've trusted these doctors to leave my cancer inside me for three months?" (So they could treat it before surgery, instead of just cutting it out like some hospitals would have.) Once we signed on at UCSF, we learned about a new kind of faith. And fear.

TRUE CONFESSION

ME: "Hmmmmm ... muhhhhh..."

PAULA: "You in pain?"

ME: "No."

Pause.

ME: "Hmmmmm ... muhhhhh ..."

PAULA: "You in denial?"

ME: "I guess so."

GOLF AND MY CANCER

Getting out of the house, putting and pitching in some cool, gray spring air at Flatirons Golf Course. Betting Jim a dollar-a-hole for closest-to-the-pin on the putting green, then swinging away, sort of, at a seventy-five yard target with a pitching wedge, aiming at a swalelike area littered with range balls.

Taking care not to take a full swing, else I may rip my implanted chest port and vein tube from their anchors under my skin by my right shoulder. Not sure whom to ask about golfing-with-a-chemo-port ... knowing that a wicked swing might send me to a hospital for unscheduled surgery.... Kinda takes the sweetness out of the short shots that I hit rather well this day.

FEAR AT THIRTY-FIVE THOUSAND FEET

Trying to forget about my disease for a few more hours as we pack up and head back to San Francisco. A week of tests, then surgery. As we hit max altitude, I pick *Parade* out of the Sunday paper and unfortunately find a story by Tad Szulc, seventy-four...a journalist who just happens to have colon cancer...that has spread unpredictably to his liver and lungs two years after surgery. "It's incurable," he writes. At this moment I am not afraid of the plane crashing. [*Editor's note: Szulc died shortly after the Parade story ran.*]

WORLD SPINNING ROUND

"I saw a lot of things spinning around my head this week," I tell Paula, trying to explain the feelings I have after yesterday's pelvic MRI, while lying on my back on a slab of hard plastic and foam, being slid, mechanically, into a chamberlike futuristic body scan, only it's not futuristic, it's now, CT-style, with unknown imaging parts spinning, whirring, racing around my body inside the machine, gaining speed and making magnetic pictures of body parts, body cavities, body systems from head to groin. And as the spin spins, a Teutonic male voice occasionally commands, and does so creepily, "Breathe in," "Hold" (for sixteen seconds yet...), "Breathe out." And again. And again. It's all prep for surgery. It's new mapping for the docs to compare with the scans they took back in January. I'm spun out.

KARMA WAVES

Waiting for Doc Daphne, the radiation doc, in Exam Room 7 of Long Hospital's basement, who's left to read the whole batch of my new films, the ones that will say how well, or not, my treatment has been going...just me and Paula sitting in the room around lunchtime with the door closed, not thinking about lunch. For what if the tumor grew during my weeks at home?

"I wish I had your karma," Doc Daphne finally says after eyeing my CTs and taking a seat next to me. Good news again; all the tests show the tumor has either shrunk or not spread. This on the very day the City of San Francisco's department of public health issues me an official plastic-coated "Medical Cannabis Voluntary ID Program" card, which will enable me to buy marijuana for medicinal uses for up to one year from today. Twenty-five dollars it cost me, plus twenty-five for Paula's card, as "caregiver," who can get the drugs if I'm laid up...or retching from chemo that's ahead. And from what I learn about the surgery today...it's going to mean laid up, or down, for at least six weeks. Bit more karma, please?

SEX AND MY CANCER [Part IV]

Taking a meeting I'd rather not take. Going to see Peter Carroll, M.D., chairman of the department of urology at UCSF, who's been asked to join my surgery team. "He's going to help me stay out of the prostate," Dr. Welton, my colorectal surgeon, says.

Stay out of the prostate indeed. It's not enough lousy luck that I—Mr. Health Book Author—get cancer, that I get colorectal cancer, that I'm going to have my abdominal organs rearranged: now one of the top urologic surgeons in the country tells me, after reviewing the MRI of my pelvis, that in surgery I may lose some of the nerves that help erections become erections. Without those nerves, bundled around the prostate and near the rectum, I understand in a hurry, I may soon be Viagra dependent, sexually speaking.

"We just want the cancer out," Paula tells Dr. Carroll. I think maybe we want a little more than that.

COUNTDOWN

T minus thirty hours and counting...till they strip me, gown me, wheel me, scrub me, shave me, drug me, prep me, cut me, eviscerate me, probe me, stimulate me (erectile nerves, that is, using a newish procedure to try to save my sexual functions), reorganize me (turning my small intestines into my small-and-large intestines and anus...), de-cancer me, maybe "muscle-flap" me (as in plastic surgery if the surgical wound gets to be tricky to close), and bring me to, as a cancer patient, as a recovering colon-cancer patient who's going to be in pain and most likely minus one colon; they're gonna do all this and more in T minus thirty hours, and I wonder why a couple of friends have asked me quite recently, "Are you nervous?" What if I said, no, I wasn't? Thing of it is, I'm going in Tuesday morning, three months after my diagnosis, six weeks after my chemo/radiation regimen; I'm going in Tuesday morning, not nervous but frightened, to get a tumor out, God and all other higher powers willing.

THE POWER OF (LEGAL) POT

Waking up one morning before dawn, with bone-numbing lower-body pain that starts me moaning-breathing-moaning and wakes up Paula. I get what the doctors mean when they say my tumor is low enough to be lodged in my pelvis. Time for narcotics, my man Vike [Vicodin], except it'll take forty-five minutes to work. We both know that by now. Which is why we have four medical joints stashed in an Altoids tin box.

"Why don't you take some pot?" Paula says.

"It's too early," I tell her. "It's not even 6:15."

A beat, then Paula responds: "It's not like you're smoking it because you don't have a job!"

I light up. It works, masking the pain without making me high, till good brother Vike kicks in.

"PLAY BALL!"

You've got to give him points for trying. My surgeon, Dr. Welton, after meeting with Paula and me to have us sign consent forms and review next week's surgery, gives us a bit of consent, too. "We've got tickets to the Giants' Opening Day—but it's the day before surgery," Paula says. "Do you think it would be okay for Curt to go?"

"Yeah," he says, knowing full well I've got to be on a liquid diet all day and take major laxatives the night before the operation. "He should be fine. As a matter of fact, I think it would be good for you guys to go.

"You can think of it this way: Monday will be baseball Opening Day and Tuesday will be our Opening Day."

This I find almost funny.

NIGHT BEFORE

"It's gonna be okay," I say to Paula with eight hours to go till surgery.

Silence.

"You know why?" I ask.

She shakes her head no.

"Because of you, because of what I have to live for," I say.

(MONTH FOUR)

Following chemo and radiation treatment, surgery was scheduled for April 3.

PRE-OP PEP TALK

"Hey," I say to Paula, after the travel alarm *chirps-chirps-chirps* us awake, "let's go get some cancer out." Sounds like I'm cheerleading on Surgery Day but I'm not. Just making light in the early-A.M. dark.

"Hey," I say, "let's go get some cancer out."

ROAD TRIP

Rolling through the pitch-black streets of San Francisco toward the hospital, our pal Aimee at the wheel, Paula up front, me stretched out at an odd angle in between the backseat; still hurts to sit straight up on my tumor.

Time to cut the vile thing from my body. Traffic at 6:30's a breeze, though I'm wishing it weren't. I'm suddenly in no hurry...thinking about the odd positions they're gonna have me in throughout this ordeal...this total colectomy or whatever. Too late to worry, but I'm wondering, still, whether the pre-op chemo/radiation combo actually shrank my tumor enough to allow these UCSF doctors to excise all of what we all want excised. Don't want to hear they got "most of it": that means I could be back here in a couple years, the "absolutely curable" me, rolling through the darkened streets once more, heading for more cancer surgery after having tried— and likely failed—to renew my six-year-old term life-insurance policy.

PRE-OP PREP WALK

As Dr. Mark Welton said last week, it's Opening Day! But before he opens me up and takes out what's evil, they've got to check me in, like at some hotel of horrors in the gloam of pre-sunrise, and they've got to have me perform a macabre march-of-the-day—with two other patients (one in a wheelchair) and a nurse in the lead, here we go!—from ground-floor check-in to pre-op anesthesia up on four.

Shuffling our way through the halls of Moffitt-Long Hospital, waiting for our appointed docs and drugs. Last time I'll be wearing street clothes for a week, I think, as I tote a large plastic "Patient Belongings" bag that now belongs to me. I look at Paula, who looks sad walking beside me; we're in the back of the pack....I feign a stop-look-and-run away from the group, like a kid on a fourth-grade field trip to some boring modern-art museum, only this ain't a museum and the only exhibit worth looking at around these parts is still lodged deep in my pelvis—call it Exhibit A. Or more accurately, Exhibit C.

CUTTING REMARKS

Can't say I saw what I'm about to say here, but if what they say is true about my operation, it didn't go well...it went better than well. I mean, "We got a better result than we even hoped for back in January," said Alan Venook, M.D., my medical oncologist. I'll take it.

I didn't see where the first scalpel started, but I do see I have an eleven-inch abdominal incision, held closed by forty-two metal staples, which artfully arcs around my belly button (doctors don't mess with belly buttons), where they "entered" and removed my entire colon and rectum (just lucky, I guess, as I've read 85 percent of colon-cancer patients don't need to have their entire colons removed—they just lose a few inches of intestine). I also feel but can't see a five-inch incision down around my anus, which means in order to excise my rectal tumor completely, they had to cut me from above and below. Not your standard, slam-dunk polyp removal, which is why the surgery took eight hours instead of two or three. [It was a stubborn rectal tumor, says Doc Welton, in retrospect. And it was, he reminds me: a newish, nerve-sparing operation...a TME, or total mesorectal excision, with which not all cancer surgeons are familiar.] There's also a newly created hole in my lower torso through which my intestines and stoma (aka my new anus) now feed.

And the good news again? Hey, they didn't need to use the fancified, intraoperative radiation machine that was on standby...and they didn't need to use the plastic surgeon to help "close" me. (He was on standby, too.) Final pathology says that the margins around the tumor were clear...which means my team done good. Very good. They grabbed thirty-one lymph nodes out of me, thirty of which were cancer-free. I'd be more worried about the one that wasn't, except that I now know at least a few other lymph nodes were probably also cancerous back in January and February...and my pre-op chemo/ radiation killed the cancer in those. Had they operated in January, I might've had six cancerous nodes and twenty-five "clean." So the single bad node doesn't worry me right now because, docs say, they got clear margins. The tumor and surrounding nodes were encapsulated. I can live with that, in more ways than one.

AN ICE PLACE TO VISIT

Welcome to the RR—recovery room—where they wheel me after the OR, where a lot happens in a hurry, in a flurry, and yet I remember only a few things:

1.that Paula was there to my right, telling me that "they...got...it...all";

2. that a nurse to my left, who was taking all sorts of measurements and checking multiple monitors and related tethers, had to leave in a hurry because her car was parked at a meter;

3. that I could...barely...breathe— felt like my chest was crushed—"Don't

worry," they said. Just the after-effects of the ventilator and my lungs being turned off for eight hours; and

4. that I was thirsty like I've never been, but the nurse wouldn't let me have water, else I might throw up, faint from the pain, and get pneumonia... "Here, have some ice chips, but don't swallow the melt...." Great Crushed ice-chip pebbles, one-at-a-time on my tongue, but Don't Swallow?? Can hardly believe it...can hardly breathe...go feed the meter....

THE RECOVERY PARADE

Watching patients outside my hospital room shuffling round the fourteenth floor—two, three, five days after major surgery—where they test their legs and upright powers. Being sort of amazed, racked with nonstop aching torso pain, that I'm soon walking beside them, even with megadoses of morphine and epidural infusions in my spine, even if in Cro-Magnon man fashion, less than seventy hours after waking up, minus one tumor and minus one colon.

CATHETER BLUES

Glad, really glad, I wasn't conscious when they shoved the rubber tube through my penis and urethra and into my bladder during surgery. Watching roller-coaster rivulets of pee move out of me every few hours. It stings sometimes; other times I shudder from terrific, searing bladder spasms after I'm done, robbing me of whatever hint of genital pleasure a "normal" good piss might provide. As my surgeon would say, "Those tissues are angry down there. They don't like what we've done to them." Neither, for the moment, do I.

THE ENDORSEMENT: THE BAG [Part I]

Leaning forward in her chair, Susan Barbour, nurse on the colorectal-surgery floor, patiently explains it all to me: how the colostomy/ileostomy bag works, the hassles and tricks, and even a fashion tip or two for when I rejoin the real world, cancer-free. "So, how do you feel about it?"

Takes a while to answer her, as I guess I have two answers. "I'm thinking about it as if I have a handicap," I say, "but a very small handicap. That's how I feel about it. Basically, I don't want my life controlled by body waste."

A FIRM FUTURE?

No way to prep for it, but two days after they pull my catheter, while peeing into a plastic urinal, I see the beginnings of an erection happening. Beginnings get all the way to middles...which makes me think they were pretty damn successful during surgery and makes me later blurt to Paula across the room: "Don't forget to tell Dr. Welton about my erection this morning."

She tells him while on the phone; I see her smile at his response. He says, "I think this might be the first time I've been so happy about another man's erection. I'll have to tell my wife about this." I'm happy and all, having seemingly dodged Viagra-dependence...but I'm still bedbound, in pain, being fed a couple bags of fluids a day...400 calories each plus ice chips—"No swallowing the melt!"—wondering, well, should he have sounded that surprised?

A "BEAUTIFUL" STOMA

Not one but two or three nurses who've viewed my carved-up body have commented on the craftsmanship of my colorectal surgeon: "A beautiful stoma," one says. "Oh, your stoma looks great," says another. "Really nice."

This does not exactly sink in. For where I used to have a flat lower right abdomen, I now have a ruddy, sturdy, slippery, inch-high plug of intestinal protrusion, a stoma they call it, a beautiful stoma they call it sometimes, a rerouting of small intestine that will serve as an anchor of sorts for the plastic bags I will fasten to my lower torso, which will collect my crap round-the-clock. I am cancer-free, with a good prognosis. And a beautiful stoma.

CURRENCY EXCHANGE

Phone rings, I pick up. It's Marsha, our friend, who's been there since Day One after diagnosis, who was there in the waiting area the day of surgery, and after....

"Hi, Curt," she says, which tells me she's back from vacation in Costa Rica. "We brought you some extra *colones*," she adds. Turns out the colon—ironically or not—is the unit of currency in Costa Rica. So maybe I should pay my surgeon with 'em?

CHEATING ON MY WIFE

Waiting for Doc Welton to come in the exam room and check his/my stitches and see how I'm doing post-op, when I spot a scale across the hall....

I strip off my jacket and step on, watching the needle on the dial spin round twice...100 pounds...then 150 and still climbing...to 164. Paula peers over my right shoulder as I shuffle my feet slightly, then some more, and watch the needle creep up to 167. I'm cheating, in full view of my wife. I want her to see me as stronger, bigger, healthier than I was on that horrid day in the hospital seven days post-op when I hardly tipped the scales at 153. Unlike cheating husbands, hospital scales don't lie.

BOX SCORE

Odds are in, two weeks after surgery, and I'm okay with them:

- I should have 70 percent of my strength back three months after surgery.

- I should have 90 percent of my strength after six months (barring complications).

- I am taking seventeen pills a day—eight of them narcotics—to relieve the pain from my operation.

- There's a better-than-60-percent chance that I'll be colon-cancer-free five years from now.

THE ENDORSEMENT: THE BAG [Part II]

It is not exactly pretty; it is something I am not exactly proud of. The bag I now wear, along with thousands of other colorectal-cancer survivors, is an opaque, white-trimmed polyethylene utensil not that different in shape or appearance from a flattened, up-side-down, old-fashioned milk bottle, the kind you see at carnivals and county fairs–three throws for a dollar...knock 'em off the table...for the big-ass stuffed animal!

The bag is two fists tall or thereabouts, reaching, as I stand, from next to my navel to the glans of my (nonerect) penis. The bag, also called "the pouch" by ostomy experts, is emptied three times a day and at bedtime and changed every three days or so. Featuring two openings—one that attaches to my lower torso with skin-friendly adhesives, the other that empties into the toilet and clips shut—the bag is a lot better alternative than an adult diaper, I'd say; others might say, cynically, "That Depends." I would not however say that. For the bag is airtight-watertight-hygienic. Even as it is not exactly attractive.

"You can wear it under your trunks while swimming," a forthright nurse tells me the other day. This I ponder for more than a minute. For I realize that my swim trunks aren't exactly attractive. Nor, on even my best days at the RallySport Health Club pool, are they something I am exactly proud of. But they do the job. So, it seems, does the bag.

SEX AND MY CANCER [Part V]

A few weeks after surgery—more than three, but who's counting?—I'm fooling around in bed with Paula, and it feels like high school fooling-around-in-bed....Because, honestly, I don't know what will happen...on my side of the bed...if we keep this up. Fact is...plumbing's been shut off for a while. Lotsa hands, more than usual, it seems. And I'm not thinking about baseball or the Queen Mother; I'm thinking, for a few seconds at least, about Peter Carroll, M.D., and his finely trimmed mustache and glasses and his ultraclean office and the meeting we had in late March, when he warned me that I might be Viagra-dependent...for a while. For a long while.

Maybe for decades...but...not...now.... "First time since surgery," I'm thinking, feeling a lot like in high school right now, with lotsa hands...and an odd, resurgent, genital-tickle-toward-inevitability...and a rhythmic pumping in the erection that almost wasn't...hold on...on the verge...of bringing unfamiliar groans of pleasure.

Feels so good I feel like shouting but I don't. Instead I'll just write about it, quietly, in the pages of a national magazine. And maybe take a nap.

POST-OP PEP TALK

"So," says my best friend, Geoff, settling in for a visit after flying himself and his family halfway across the country to see me soon after surgery, "lemme see the bag."

He's not talking lost luggage from the flight. He means the bag that holds my poo.

"Okay," I say, knowing he'd ask, "but first drop your pants and bend over." He doesn't laugh. Or drop trou.

"You've seen one before," he says.

"Not yours," I say.

He smiles: "I guess they're the same thing, huh?"

Guess so.

SURGICAL STRIKE

Three weeks ago today, a couple of doctors I knew, and eight of whom I didn't, gathered in the OR of Moffitt Hospital to put me under, take me apart, and put me back together. They gathered that Tuesday in April to try to make me a patient who used to have cancer. They gathered to take on a disease that grew for years by division-cell division—and yet the success of their surgery would hinge on collaboration.

There would be no room for error, really. A strike in baseball—"*Steeee-rii-iike!!!*"—means a pitcher's hit his target A successful surgical strike in cancer-speak means They Got It All, with "clear margins." Turns out the sonsaguns done committed a successful surgical strike, oncologically speaking. Sonsagun surgeons, Dr. Mark Lane Welton and Dr. Peter Carroll, came strutting down the hall after eight hours of tough surgery on my body and my malignancy; sonsaguns came down the hall in their surgical blues, smiling like they'd done roped the biggest mean-ol' steer at the state fair ro-de-o. I'd tip my ten-gallon to 'em, but I'm still unconscious, waiting to wake up in the recovery room and hear Paula repeat what the doctors told me but I did not hear: that I am cancer-free. For now at least; hopefully, till the day I die. Of other causes. Sonsaguns hit the mitt.

(MONTH FIVE)
Following treatment and surgery, post-op chemotherapy began on schedule.

POST-OP PROGNOSIS [Part I]

ESTABLISHING SHOT: *Helicopter cam pans south from Golden Gate Bridge and yacht-infested Marina to the cluster of medical buildings crammed into a hill beneath Twin Peaks....*

INTERIOR: *Sixth-floor exam room, Surgery Faculty Practice Building, University of California, San Francisco, 400 Parnassus Avenue.*

"We couldn't have been happier with the way [surgery] went," says Doc Welton, my trusty colorectal surgeon. But when I ask half kiddingly, "Then why do we need to do chemo?" he mentions the possibilities of microscopic cells left behind that could mean Big Trouble later.

"We're trying to predict the behavior of a tumor, and we can't do that yet," Doc Welton says. It seems even the most successful surgery can't account for pre-cancerous cells too small to be seen. So then, chemo-time to be safe.

SYNOPSIS: *Surgery a success; so too the pre-op radiation and chemo. Still, they're gonna hook me up and infuse me; they're gonna burn the village to save the village.*

F-U

Listening intently as Dr. Venook lays it out forthrightly a few days before my first big IV blast. "We use two drugs in combination," he says. One they've already pumped into my body before surgery, 5-fluorouracil (5-FU—or just "F-U" to colon-cancer veterans), and leucovorin, an acid, a cousin to folic acid, that helps the 5-FU do its thing. I'm doing my best to consider this course of chemo "preventive." Just can't wait for side effects like vomiting, nausea, hair loss, weight loss, infection. You know, minor things when compared with "locally invasive" cancer like I had... Still, I'm not breathing too easily…"There's a third drug that some centers were experimenting with," Venook adds, "but three deaths were recently reported in clinical trials." We'll stick with the first two drugs then.

[Note: see pg. 110 for updated chemo/biotherapy regimens]

DOWN-AND-UP

Getting tired of the post-op routine: two hours down, forty-five minutes up, waiting for my abdomen muscles, anal stitches, and innards to heal…. Can't sit yet. Comfortably, that is. Couple hours of work, a meal here, a meal there, some TV….

Two weeks out of the hospital and I'm still, basically, horizontal. Or walking, slowly, sorta upright. It's a start.

CALL IT SMACKEY

Waking up one morning in week four of chemo with a small pool of metallic saliva on the back of my tongue. Saliva's telling me my body—my bone marrow actually—has been thoroughly invaded by the 5-FU and is On the Case. Not quite sick enough to throw up; not quite strong enough to shake it off and pretend I'm gonna have a great day. It's a minor part of the assault, unpleasant and tenacious, that attacks my tongue three, four times a week, four, five hours a day, sending copperesque spittle down my gullet; reminding me that I'm still a patient under treatment at an NIH-designated comprehensive cancer center and that more than a few mornings during the rest of my May-June regimen, I will wake up feeling like crap.

The feeling makes me smack my tongue to the roof of my mouth—once, twice, thrice....[My wife] Paula now knows the sound and what it means. Call it smackey, she says. So I do. And suck on a butterscotch, to *beat smackey down.*

THE METALLIC-MOUTH DIET

First thing chemo does some days is mess with the taste buds. There are days when I can't eat fish, chicken, meat, eggs, greens, tomato sauce, or hot *anything* without feeling sick.

Today, like many days, Haagen-Dazs is my dinner.

MAGIC FINGERS

Watching as our friend and massage therapist, James, walks into the living room lugging his fold-up, fold-out table, getting ready to set up and work on Paula's and my dad's stressed and sore backs.

Knowing full well that I could use, at this point of my recovery, something approximating a friendly, warm touch, but, truth is, I don't want anybody touching me, not now, not for a while; for I have been touched, poked, stuck, burned, inspected, opened, rearranged, closed, and inspected some more by so many strangers and almost-strangers in the last three months that my mind tells my body not to trust anyone not married to me whose fingers and hands want to get close to me. For now, three weeks after surgery, it's all too much. And I recoil: No touching, not yet.

SURGEON SPEAK

Today Doc Welton tells me, at four weeks post-op (after I complain about feeling trapped indoors): "That's how you know you're getting better: When you start getting ticked off about not being able to get out and do things, you're healing." Yeah, right.

WHO IS THIS WOMAN LYING NEXT TO ME?

Because of my surgery, because of my drugs, I cannot write the three paragraphs that follow. I'll need a little help (once again) from my wife, this time from her journal.

Sometimes Curt's memory is foggy. No, actually his memory is sometimes gone. If he acted goofy I might expect it, but he looks me in the eyes, smiles, and agrees to something and then later doesn't recall the conversation ever took place. (Apparently, after you have an eight-hour surgery, anesthesia, chemo, and are taking long-term narcotics for pain, your short-term memory takes a beating.)

It's hard for me to believe that Dr. Welton stood at the foot of Curt's bed telling him, "After seeing your tumor, I'm convinced it was at least eight to ten years old." Later, I hear Curt telling a friend about his "five-year-old tumor." I tell him what Dr. Welton had said about it being eight to ten years old, and he looks at me completely shocked and asks, "Did he really say that? When?"

People show up at our door that I'm not expecting and who have called to ask if I need anything because they're on their way. Lately Curt has been forgetting phone calls. Or parts of calls. Out of character. Because of this, I'm afraid for Curt to go to any doctor appointments alone. I'm there to mentally record the conversations, just in case. I am told by Dr. Welton that the forgetfulness is completely normal and shouldn't last more than a year. Curt looks at me every night and tells me he loves me; that I know—but is he really talking to me?

POST-OP PROGNOSIS [Part II]

INTERIOR: *Darkened bedroom, 5:30 a.m., camera push [wife's POV] into husband rolling slowly out of bed.*

CUT TO: *Int. bathroom dimly lit, mirror shot reveals husband standing in front of toilet with doughnut-sized ring of pee on Calvin Klein boxers.*

Son...of...a... body, don't break down on me now ...waking up at dawn to pee, easing my aching body, face up, off the bed into upright position with strategic use of elbow power and knee leverage (I look and feel like a damn Dungeness crab), and flicking on the bathroom light: Something's wrong. There, on my gray cotton underwear, to the right of where my penis resides, is a spot, a wet spot, bigger than a quarter, a lot bigger than a quarter. My eyes lock in on the spot, or rather the reflection of the spot in the bathroom mirror. I don't believe it: After what I've been through, from life-threatening diagnosis through chemo/radiation, bone-racking pain to setbacks and major, life-saving surgery, now I've got to suffer the indignity of a leaking hose?

Not quite twelve hours later, my surgeons have slipped me into their schedules to see what's up, bladderwise. Did they nick a urogenital nerve somewhere during surgery? No time to ponder possibilities I have no clue about; it's time to piss into a "Flowmeter" contraption in the urology clinic, a spinning disc beneath a large funnel, set up atop a toilet that measures urine volume and force of the stream. These are things I've never had checked before, as I'm not a seventy-eight-year-old with prostate troubles. But I whip it out, hit the target, and watch a needle record my output.

Then it's flush, wash up, and hop over to the ultrasound room, where Nurse Dora squirts cold jelly on my belly—"Watch the incision stitches," I plead—and starts pressing on me with a wand as she looks for the grainy shadows of my bladder on screen. Seems at first glance I'm "emptying okay"; seems that my stop/start mechanisms of urination are in working order as well. For now, docs think the trouble's not uromechanical but actually a side effect: As I'm still healing from the surgery, still popping seventeen pain pills round the clock, I'm sleeping "better," longer, more soundly, than I've slept in months. And as the pain eases each week, the narcotics apparently put me under so deeply that I don't feel the first inner twinges of taking a piss that normally would wake me. After all, docs point out, the urine leaking ain't happening during the day when I'm awake (as it does with many prostate-cancer patients)....

Feeling better now about half of my excretionary equipment, feeling that even though my colon and rectum were removed, maybe I won't need bladder surgery to fix my powers of urination. Unfortunately, I'm supposed to make a follow-up appointment. Unfortunately I'll be back.

SYNOPSIS: *Seems to me, if life were fair, a recovering cancer patient who craps in a bag shouldn't have to worry about a leaky dick.*

SEX AND MY CANCER [Part VI]

Stumbling upon the startling statement in a "Chemotherapy and You" brochure: "It is advisable to wear a condom during intercourse for up to 48 hours after treatment, as chemotherapy drugs may be present in sperm," and at once being taken aback and frightened. For me and for Paula, who I may be unwittingly poisoning. "Nobody told me this," I'm thinking, while hurriedly doing the math. I breathe easier when it computes: It's been at least seventy-two hours since my last dose of chemo. So last night was okay. In more ways than one.

DR. WORTHLESS...
STLL COMPLETELY WORTHLESS

Phone rings. Paula answers. It's Dr. Fuller, her OB-GYN, calling from Denver to see how we're doing...it reminds me that he's called four times since my diagnosis, and my ex-gastro, Dr. Worthless, who missed what they now think was an eight-to-ten-year-old rectal tumor three and a half years ago during a screening colonoscopy, hasn't called since December. Reminds me also of the two visits I made to Worthless last summer and fall, complaining of rectal pain each time but not receiving a basic, digital rectal exam either time.

All this sends me to the Net, to a leading malpractice lawyer's Web site and then further...where I soon learn Dr. Worthless's Colorado medical board "license status" is "active" and also learn that there is "no disciplinary information on file."

Not yet, anyway.

POT LUCK

In my left hand, I hold a plastic card that has my picture on it, a card issued by the San Francisco Department of Public Health. It reads: "Medical Cannabis Voluntary Identification Program. Issue Date: 29-Mar-01; Expires: 29-Mar-02." I use this card when making legal purchases. In my right hand, I hold a newspaper clipping, front-page story, of the *San Francisco Chronicle* that reads: MEDICINAL POT RULED ILLEGAL

In my recent memory, I hold an image of me, lying on our couch, moaning in severe pain, arms at my side, fists clenched, kicking my legs in staccato spasms, trying to send the pain from a stage-3 tumor lodged in my pelvis out of my body and out of my mind.

In my not-so-recent memory, I hold an image of me driving a car, cocking my head in disbelief at a proposed Supreme Court Justice, Clarence Thomas, in a Senate hearing in D.C, being accused by a college law professor, Anita Hill, of sexually harassing her in part by telling her he found a pubic hair atop a can of Coca-Cola that was on his desk. I wondered then, What could he possibly have been thinking?

In my left hand, I hold a recent weekly newspaper clipping from a wire service that says Clarence Thomas found that "medical necessity is not a defense to manufacturing and distributing marijuana." I wonder now, halfway through chemo, What could he possibly be thinking?

DERAILED

"Once you've been hit by the train so many times," Paula tells me in bed this morning, "you're afraid to stand on the tracks to see if another one's coming." No wonder my wonderful wife is scared at this point in my treatment...it's time to schedule the first series of "follow-up" CT scans. We know the drill: head, chest, abdomen, pelvis. Send some ultra-energy X-ray beams through my organs and bones and see what shows up on film....

"...so many times..." Paula saying about the train makes me think: I've been hit once—and good—by the Colorectal Express...whereas she recalls, and for good reason, five derailments:

- 1994, her niece, our niece, Sandra, getting hit by a logging truck on a Sierra mountain road, falling into a coma for fourteen months, and still recovering from brain damage seven years later....

- 1994, her brother, Larry, falling thirty feet off a roof on a house he was painting, landing facedown and surviving, being medevacked and plastic-surgically put back together, one facial bone at a time....

- 1997, suffering a life-threatening ruptured ectopic pregnancy that sent her tumbling to the floor and into surgery while her blood pressure read an absolutely mind-numbing 50/0. (I didn't even know you could have zero BP and survive....)

- 1999, while out of town on a job, finding a lump in her throat, lodged deeply in her thyroid, causing docs to operate and me to forever associate driving across the Golden Gate Bridge, alone, into San Francisco, with heading to the hospital to get her post-op results from pathology. TGIB, Thank God It's Benign, we were able to say....

And, hey, not to worry for a while...till December 2000, when that last frickin' choo-choo decided to derail me, her, both of us, I guess, which is why I might be a little more scared of those upcoming CTs, come to think of it, than I'm letting on. Even though they come back negative for cancer, I'll always need to be prepared for The Next Scan.

HALFWAY HOME?

Flipping the page on the calendar, saying so long to May, seeing how many days we have left in San Francisco—for treatment and packing—and focusing on June 17. Then it's home to Denver/Boulder for final chemo and settling back in.

Got the diagnosis in late December; started treatment in early January. Got six weeks of radiation/chemo in January and February, rad burns finally healed in late March.

Got operated on in early April in a major way; finally healed in—what am I talking about, it's early June and I still haven't "finally" healed. Can't even roll all the way over in bed, for the cut stomach muscles that still ache daily and deeply.

Got six weeks of chemo in May and June; have six more to go before I flip the calendar past July and August. Somehow, by my count, feels like I am only halfway home. Go figure.

CHEMO-BY-THE-BAY

Easing into a leatherette La-Z-Boy in the UCSF infusion center, waiting for my blood work and for two friends to come by. (Farley's a San Fran local; Pete'll fly in from Denver for a few hours.) Suddenly I hear Paula say, "Oh, my God, there's Brandy!"—meaning my grade-school friend who's joined by my high-school bud Jerry, which means we're having a surprise San Francisco-chemo-by-the-Bay party, only half of which I was expecting....

Can't believe these guys pulled this one off—that with four wives and thirteen kids among them, they were able to shuck their schedules, blow off clients, and see if they couldn't give me some old-style, are-we-ever-gonna-grow-up, ball-busting support. On a day I might not feel much like partying.

For the occasion, Farley rents a 1450cc Harley (which Brandy falls off of while stopped at a stoplight); Pete raids the free (!) graham-crackers-and-apple-juice "for patients only" pantry; and Jerry makes gross jokes about the rubber gloves he doesn't seem to want to take off....I'm back in high school again, laughing my ass off with old friends ...till the drugs make me weak and the airport calls the boys home.

(MONTH SIX)

UNTIED

There are days, many days after surgery, that I don't tie my shoes because it hurts too much to bend over. So I tuck the laces under the tongue, making my cross-trainers into loafers, and spare myself the indignity of asking my wife to help me make a bow.

262,800 MINUTES

Packing up, in our friends Monica's and Chris's home, packing up to go home. Half a year we've lived out of town, or 262,800 minutes if you go by the lyrics of *Rent*, which we saw at the Orpheum the other night. "How do you measure, measure a year?"

Six months of diagnoses and treatment and recoveries and there are still six weeks of chemo sessions left, which I'll get in Denver, under the guidance of my San Fran doctors. Call it aftercare, even if it isn't quite. And if anything should go wrong, really or terribly wrong, I'll be back in San

Francisco quick as United Air can take me, for there's a trust I'm not yet willing to share. All these minutes later.

214,600 DOLLARS

Filing the bills that have found us at home, sent from all of the parties who have played a part in my cancer assault. Wondering if and when we're gonna hit the $300,000 mark in assessed billings.

BREAST CANCER AND MY CANCER

Can't stop 'em, but good friends and colleagues are talking to me more about cancer these days, breast cancer and colon cancer mostly, diseases that seem to bring extraordinary surprise to others when they learn of diagnoses that have hit people close to them.

"You're not supposed to get breast cancer at forty-four," or thirty-eight, or whatever, I hear. Same goes for colon cancer or rectal cancer. There's some bond there; as a friend of mine put it, "It's the f---ed-upness of a young person getting cancer." Then there's the follow-up f'd-upness of radiation or chemo or both and maybe some kind of mental bluesy funk when all the bad cells have been exterminated.

There's something else, too: the fact that I worked for seven years for the women's magazine that started the Pink Ribbon Breast Cancer Awareness Campaign. I'm an unlikely cancer vet. I used to write about breast cancer without feeling truly close to it. I can now relate to cancer patients in ways that I couldn't before...whether I like it or not. It's different to talk about it and to write about it...than to have it.

TOUGH DAY, DUDE

Strolling out of chemo, glad to have another blast out of the way, walking up to the car, and staring, blankly, at the windshield. Great. Guy goes into the esteemed Rocky Mountain Cancer Center to try to kick cancer's ass; meantime some fake-cop parking jockey sees I've been in there for more than two hours, slaps us with a fifteen-buck ticket.

Didn't we see *the sign?*

Tough day, dude.

A WORSE PERSON?

I used to be a happy guy. People say I've always been happy. Haven't felt that way in a while and instead feel that I'm not as nice a person as I used to be. Question is, why am I now less tolerant of other people? Especially after getting tons of support from my family, friends, and incredibly kind strangers. "It's not just getting cancer," Paula says. "It's the threat of get- ting cancer, facing death, your mortality, that's made you different. You don't have patience for insincerity anymore. Once your security and hap- piness are threatened, you can't be the same." But am I worse?

UNFORGIVEN

While pondering a suit in Denver against my former gastroenterologist, I'm not thinking big $ at all. Hell, I now know (but didn't know three months ago) there's a $1 million medical-malpractice cap in Colorado.

And I know he didn't give me cancer. But the way I see it, the doctor I'm thinking of suing did not practice good medicine upon me. Not even "acceptable" medicine upon me.

He scoped me in '97, missed some advanced rectal cancer (according to another doctor whom I do respect); then failed to perform a digital rectal exam twice when I went to him complaining of rectal pain. When I got my rectal-cancer diagnosis from him in December, I was stunned. Then I got angry. Six months later, whether or not I end up going forward with a lawsuit, he's still unforgiven.

HATE LETTERS

Never heard the phrase spoken to me till I got cancer and then got rid of it. Never heard a doctor say, "I get at least a couple of hate letters every year," especially a doctor of mine [Dr. Alan Venook, my oncologist] who's committed to serving patients who now have or have had cancer. Sticks in my mind: "...a couple of hate letters every year." For telling people news they didn't, or don't, want to hear; for telling people they have cancer, and for sometimes telling people they have cancer and that they don't have that many options to fight it. Which means there's a lot of pain going round these halls. And a few painful letters in answer to a new kind of pain. Hate letters, the doctor says. I decide to send the guy a nice note.

INSOMNIAC ADDICT

Padding about the bedroom and kitchen in moccasin-slippered feet, in search of Cheerios and milk, wondering what this buzz in my veins could possibly mean, this unfocused energy that's been keeping me up till 3:00 a.m. for days now, or for nights, rather, as my pain subsides and my trip through chemoland begins to feel commonplace.

Thinking to myself (who else would be up at this hour?) that maybe I've been taking too many narcotics lately.

Figuring out, when I wake all groggy and disheveled, fogged-in and angry-tired at 9:00 a.m., feeling like I've been partying or drinking the night before...figuring out that because I've been taking the narcotic Vicodin for pain for five and a half months now and cut the dose by 90 percent over the past ten days, I'm somehow going through a skittish-sleepless withdrawal.

I've taken Vikes at bedtime since December for cancer and surgery pain—and check with Dr. Mark Welton [my surgeon] the next day about my theory. He doesn't seem worried at all when he says, "Technically, you're addicted. But that doesn't mean you'll be an addict."

I've got to taper down more slowly, he says, and might even still take a Vike at night for a while, until I begin to heal more to the point where I can move around without pain and can physically tire myself out...and so to sleep.

But not at this moment, in the dark hours between 2:00 and 4:00 a.m. on a Monday that's not starting out well. I'm hooked, for the time being. I'm an up-all-night, cancer-free, recovering colon-cancer patient who now has another health problem with which to concern himself.

CHEMO-BY-THE-ROCKIES

Chemo blows. It's "toxic medicine" to some, wickedly effective for others. It's methodically pumped into my veins by a Sigma infusion pump that has a "syringe holder" feature and an "air upstream occlusion" alarm. The chemo finds its way into the bone marrow, and that's why its kick is so powerful.

I have the flu. But not quite. I've started another chemotherapy session (my third six-week course), and I am nauseated for at least a few hours, sometimes up to eight or ten hours a day. But I don't have the flu, not quite, and I don't throw up. If I were a guy who paid no mind to post-feminist culture, I'd liken my nausea to that suffered in the early terms of pregnancy...except...here I am taking electro-pumped poison to kill some potentially malignant cells that would kill me if I didn't try to fight them.

But I'm fighting what I can't feel and what the doctors can't see or guarantee is still there—microscopic precancerous cells in my body. The stuff may work; in reality it does quite often. Nonetheless, chemo blows.

WEED...BE...GONE

Bending down in the backyard, still moving in slow-mo postsurgical fashion, to grab hold of a dandelion-gone-beanstalk in the raised garden bed, to take back some of the earth that's gone wild with weedy growths since we've been off fighting some cancer in San Francisco....

Ripping out some grass as I yank the weed in my gloved right hand, taking out more dirt than I intend to, flashing back to the talk I had with Doc Welton after my surgery: "What does it feel like to take out tumor?" I ask, invoking some faux O.R.-speak. "You cut—and then pull," he answers. "You cut tension. It's like pulling sod up from the ground...you pull a 'corner' till it's taut, then cut, then pull some more, and cut away at the point of tension."

Okay, then, when you're a colorectal surgeon like Welton, you don't take tumor timidly. "In my residency," he tells me later, "I had one chief [resident] who told me, when you're operating on a cancer patient and he's open from above, you don't stop cutting till you see the table." Don't know why the good doc shared that one with me—on second thought, I'd asked him. And the tension part hits home. I grab the next Mr. Evil Weed, dig my fingers down, and pull down below ground line. I pull like someone who's decidedly not feeling sorry for wayward greenery today. I get it out, root and all, and toss it in the pile that'll end up in the thirty-gallon Cinch Sak Hefty Bag...no need to send that sucker to pathology.

A DOZEN WORDS ABOUT DEATH

Oddly, I feel no closer to death than I did last December.

3:47 A.M.

Waking up wired, after going to bed wired, "addicted" or "Vicodin-dependent"—who gives a shit what it's called—any which way, it feels like two dozen bees are buzzing in my chest, shoulders, and arms...and suddenly I have empathy for Matthew Frickin' Perry, for chrissakes. Doc Welton says it could take weeks to kick; Doc Venook concurs. Doc Cohn [Dr. Allen Cohn, my new oncologist in Denver] talks up Benadryl a bit. Paula wants to feed my face nocturnally to get me through this withdrawal.

This is great: Try OTC antihistamines; feed the bees. But all I want is some z's.

POST-OP PROGNOSIS [Part III]

INTERIOR: *Harshly lit windowless exam room #10, Rocky Mountain Cancer Center, Denver. Paula's POV of Dr. Allen Cohn palpating my torso with his fingers.*

CUT TO: *Closeup of Dr. Cohn's face, looking unconcerned, as his circling index and middle fingers stop on my chest, upper right quadrant.*

"This mole needs to come off," he says.

CUT TO: *My face looking seemingly unconcerned.*

"I've had that checked before," I say.

CUT TO: *Paula's face, looking concerned.*

CUT TO: *3-Shot, push-in to Dr. Cohn.*

"I'd feel better if it were in a jar," Dr. Cohn says.

SYNOPSIS: *In less than three weeks, it will be. I'm going to have a new dermatologist. It's never too soon to prevent cancer.*

THE CELEBRITY OF CANCER

"They say that people who go through stuff like you've been through," an ex-colleague writes, "have a profoundly changed perspective on life—that surviving something like this can paradoxically make you a happier person than you were before. Any truth to this?"

Hell if I know.

I didn't ask to be Cancer Boy....I certainly didn't audition. But I have been feeling increasingly weird over the past six months, not just physically but about how people treat me, at times making me seem like a B-list celebrity.

It's almost freakish. That because of my biology—and the anti-cancer assault that was thrown at it—people act like in some way I might be closer to God. I've been into the fire—and come back. Maybe they think I've gone into the fire for them, or, rather, instead of them. Some people say I'm brave, but let's be frank here, I didn't walk into the fire willingly. I am not exalted. Any time you do something out of the ordinary, people want to get closer to you. Thing is, this comes at a time when I typically feel like crap a few hours a day, and all I want sometimes is distance— from just about everybody.

GETTING MY LIFE BACK

Kicked my cup-a-day coffee habit through the first two rounds of chemo and didn't seem to miss it. But I've started up again at home, maybe trying to make things the same as before....

Unfroze the health-club membership in July, even though my weight lifting's restricted, trying to make me as strong as before....

Got used to waking up same time as Paula every day for months, when I needed her caregiving more; now I wake up earlier most days, same as before....Got our dog, Bolder, back the other day, chauffeured in from Chicago in the backseat of my folks' car, trying to make things nearly the same as before....It's one thing to have your life handed back to you by your doctors; it's quite another to get that life back same as before.

A BETTER PERSON?

Dropping down out of the clouds, touching down on a sunbaked runway near our Colorado home, I am happy/sad/half-healed/scared. For now, I am 912 miles away from the doctors who saved my life. I am grateful. I am healthy, after twenty-some weeks of cancer treatment and extraordinarily successful surgery. I am, again, in a position where I can say I have my life ahead of me. But am I a better person?

I've read Joyce Wadler's book, *My Breast*, in which she emerges on the back side of her cancer treatment a better woman than when she first got her gloomy biopsy results in New York City. I've read Lance Armstrong's best-seller, *It's Not About the Bike*, about his testicular cancer, recovery, and post-op Tour de France glory. Amazingly, he writes that knowing what he knows now, if he had to choose between having cancer and winning the Tour de France, he'd choose cancer. He's now a better guy. I've heard Eric Davis of the San Francisco Giants on the radio, talking about his bout with colon cancer and how it's so curable when caught early. He may be a better person, but let's be honest: He's hitting all of .198 heading into August. So many cancer-recovery stories end with an upbeat notion. That's understandable. That's admirable even. But too many of these stories end with the notion that somehow, through all the pain, their cancer has made them "a better person." This one won't.

CHAPTER 2

Putting Cancer in its Place

There's no easy way to say it, because cancer isn't easy: After all that's been thrown at us, one of the toughest challenges for any cancer patient is to move on, to trade in our medical status, to stop being a patient and start being a former patient. No matter what the pathology reports say about "clear margins" (or not exactly clear), the idea of cancer in our bodies Does Not Leave. Sure, there may be no more daily doc visits or phone calls. No weekly "bloods." No more sessions hooked up to the auto-chemo pump-on-wheels. All good. But by extension there's also a tremendous loss of support once treatment has wound down. What do you do? Now that you're *normal* again? You wait a few years, hopefully, then a couple more. You do this until maybe the 5-year mark, when you're officially, medically "cured." This is a long flippin' time.

> " Cancer's very overrated. I'm just glad I got it out of the way while I was still young. "

— Sam Taylor-Wood, at 35, prize-winning British artist and colon/breast cancer survivor

At the same time this transition is surely not as physically tough as radiation or chemotherapy. And it's not nearly as nerve-searing painful as what you felt when your tumor was first treated. Still, there's no easy way to say it because there's no easy way to do it: How do you shrink the heavy, mindful space that cancer has introduced in your day-to-day thinking, for weeks or months at a time? The fear was—and is—so real. Mortality made itself known, ahead of schedule, in your life, in your house. (Survivors know this stat too well: about 50,000 people die of colorectal cancer in the U.S. each year, or enough to fill the seats of New York's Yankee Stadium).

So when it comes to handling these haunting fears, it turns out there's a huge difference between putting cancer behind you and putting cancer "in its place." For countless numbers of my fellow survivors agree: We will never completely put it behind us. It's part of who we are as long as we live. We can, however, with some time and help, put it in a reasonable, psychological space. (I'll not soon forget the oncology nurse at UCSF who once told me, maybe a month too soon, "You're gonna' have to deal with the Bogey Man in the closet for the rest of your life," she said. "The trick is to figure out how wide you're gonna decide to leave the door open each day.") Um, okay.... The rest of this chapter looks at how patients like me, and you, and caregivers, actually do that. It's a psychological bind patients don't often talk about, at least not often enough. They see managing their cancer emotions, as I did after a nine-month treatment and surgery protocol a few years ago, as another burden. If you acknowledge you "still" have daily, weekly, whatever thoughts about recurrence, you're being honest, yes. But at the same time you're then succumbing to certain fears. And nobody wants to think about themselves as weak at a time when they are expected, rather suddenly and by so many others, to Be Strong.

Unlike the key two-year mark that colon cancer patients first set in their sights (because "of all the people who have recurrences, 80 percent of those will develop within the first two years," says Allen Cohn, M.D., of Rocky Mountain Cancer Centers in Denver), the precise time at which patient becomes ex-patient isn't in any of the medical books. It's amorphous: could be one month, or 2.5 years; and it could be never. It's tricky for patients or loved ones to wrap their arms around, even in the most treatable cases. And for most that relatively peaceful feeling doesn't arrive quickly enough.

RE-INTRO, RE-ENTRY

In my case, the time after post-op was a bit jittery. As I wrote in my journal after I'd left the hospital worlds: "Two years since diagnosis, and I am cancer free. Don't call myself a survivor…yet; feels too early. Don't call myself a 'warrior,' either. That's for the charity-fund appeal and pink-ribbon ad-campaign writers. But I've taken nine months of radiation ('We're gonna pound you,' my radiation doc said); recovered from life-saving surgery with most of my body intact; adopted a child; and I have started hugging my family and friends a bit harder.

"Call me middle-aged guy in remission—make that recovery—because the way I see it, remission means merely temporary absence of disease. Call me healthy but wary. Been bouncing back and forth from the U.S. to London, where Paula is once again working as associate producer on the *Harry Potter* films. Been writing again, even some new kinds of stuff for a TV documentary I'm trying to get made. Been getting used to getting cancer behind me, even if it'll always seem ahead of me. Also been getting used to being a new dad, to giving all sorts of care at all hours to Baby Josh, kind-of-like Paula did for me. Still don't feel, though, that beating advanced colon cancer has made me a 'better man.' Even if I am, I've noticed, more apt to sign off letters, cards and notes with 'love.' "

Paula, by contrast, didn't see me as "healthy but wary" at this juncture. I looked in her journal (with her permission, I swear) and found she's already sort-of-told me how I was putting cancer in its place:

"HE'S LIVIN'"

"Back in England, I find I'm living with a forty-four year old teenager. Curt won't be where he doesn't want to be, or with who he doesn't want to be with. He's spontaneous and seizing the moment, not wasting time with small talk, pretending he's interested. He went to a play on a whim on Friday...'*Rent*' (again)...with some college kids he didn't know who had an extra cheap ticket to spare. He ran into them in Leicester Square. I tell him I was worried. Couldn't reach him for hours. "I'm livin'! he said, and thank God he is."

THREE TIMES A YEAR

Less than three months later Paula told how *she's* putting cancer in its place. Or trying to....

"I'm in a lot better place now, I guess because it's January. Next scans aren't till the end of April. That's because Dr. Cohn says, 'CTs every three to four months (for the first two years after surgery; then every six months).' And Curt's figured out, if we stretch it out till four, that's one less per year, plus less radiation from the scans.

"I find myself now living my life with this benchmark. So far relieved, and filled with joy, but as the weeks pass, feeling the dread that slowly creeps up on me, as the next trip home gets closer. When we sit in the oncologist's office, trying to anticipate and read into his every expression...hearts-are-racing...then learning he hasn't read them yet; he'll be right back.... Trying to hear the pace of his footsteps as he returns to see if they will give me any insight as to the news about to be delivered: Do we get to continue our lives as they are—so full of love and joy, and our new baby, Joshua...or do we put on our gear again and go into to the fire and fight for life?"

"I DON'T WANNA TALK ABOUT IT"

In the mid-1990s, Judy Webster, 57, of Omaha, Nebraska, survived a diagnosis of advanced colon cancer. It was only after she'd had emergency surgery and mostly healed that she realized people of all stripes—even family members—weren't at all comfortable talking about…the certain kind of cancer that she'd had. The one that attached to her bowels.

"In 1996, people didn't talk about colon cancer," Webster says. "When I left the hospital I felt very alone. No one reached out to me, like they do for breast cancer patients [today]. The nurses were very kind, but when I went home…that was it. I just felt really alone; my cancer was not talked about. If you [walked and] went around somebody, they would just stare at you." Imagine, trying to re-enter a family situation, as it was, and being stared at, because of the *kind* of cancer you've suffered. "I do have a handful of friends that were more open. But friends, my husband's co-workers, they were afraid to say anything to me. Nowadays, there's a better understanding of it. There's openness; more education. And more understanding by the general public. So now they'll know, and maybe be able to say, 'Hey, you have colon cancer, that doesn't mean you're going to die.' When I got out of the hospital, it was like breast cancer was [considered] thirty years ago—just was not talked about at all…now it's okay to talk about it."

Not only is it 'okay' to talk about today, it turns out this kind of talk may even hold some partly-understood, powerful health and longevity benefits. According to David Spiegel, M.D., of Stanford University Medical Center in Palo Alto, California, who has studied cancer patients and talk therapy for more than 15 years, certain research trials have shown that cancer and ex-cancer patients who join support groups and "download" stresses and fears (also, joys) in group settings tend to fair better, survival-wise, than similar patients who have tended to go it alone. An important note, however, needs to be mentioned: As perhaps exciting as Dr. Spiegel's and colleagues' work has appeared, this is an *observed* relation between longevity and group therapy. It has not been proven that talk therapy is *responsible* for the increases in longevity that have been reported.

"Helping people handle the stress of cancer can help patients live longer," claims Dr. Spiegel, a world-renown clinician. "Such help includes expressive group therapy, building bonds with other [patients] in the same situation, expressing their emotions, detoxifying dying, using self-hypnosis for pain, and reordering their priorities in life."

HOW DIFFERENT ARE YOU NOW?

Although I had only been to a handful of cancer support group sessions when I started writing this book, I felt, at times, that writing about my case in a national magazine a few years earlier gave me some of the advantages of being in a group. It became, over time, therapeutic for me to "vent" on paper and onscreen. When I started writing about how cancer felt, however, I didn't know why I did it. As a writer it simply felt normal. (In a similar, more visually artistic vein, the British photographer and videographer, Sam Taylor-Wood, made a quite remarkable picture two years after her colon cancer treatment and immediately after her treatment for breast cancer. It is entitled: "Self Portrait as a Tree," and is as beautiful as it is haunting.) In addition, through writing about my case I felt some of the support-group "lift" without having made an actual link with a Colorado-based group my first year home. All the while, friends and others kept peppering me with questions about healing that helped me maybe more than I knew at the time. Such as:

"Are you doing okay? And, "What do you think caused it?"

"I don't know," I've said, in answer to both questions, at different times. What I know is I've now lived years with cancer (without even knowing it), and a few years with a body that can be called "cancer-free." I don't believe I am "happier" than I was five years ago. But I'm beginning to put cancer in its place; for now, that means not quite behind me. Which seems normal, at least to me.

NOT EXACTLY NORMAL

"My life will never be whatever normal is," says Lisa Dubow, 47, of Los Angeles, a Stage IV patient who has surprised–time and again–teams of researchers with her resilience and healing abilities since her diagnosis and first treatments in 2001. "It wasn't normal before, but this gives me more passion to become active, to give me more time to be more politically active, and the joy of seeing a change in my life." When Dubow talks about political activism, for her that means health activism more so than traditional Democrat/ Republican U.S. politics. Specifically, she is a state coordinator for the Colon Cancer Alliance in Southern California.

"And to be honest," Dubow says, "I've actually guided people [toward research trials, new drugs]. I'm not a doctor, but I've guided people to certain doctors; I have saved certain people's lives, and it's awesome."

[Editor's note: Advocate Lisa Dubow passed away in July, 2007]

The more I've talked with patients and their families, the more I've found we aren't all afraid to shed our formerly protective habits. This is a tough transition for some; a bit less so for others…. Talking about colon cancer surely wasn't easy, at first, for someone like Katie Couric, of NBC's *Today* show, who has mobilized millions of dollars—and people—in support of colon cancer awareness since her late husband, Jay Monahan, died at age 42 of the disease in 1998. Couric even went so far as to broadcast her own colonscopy on morning television in 2000, as part of Colorectal Cancer Awareness Month. (In fact, a few years later she told a press conference audience that her colonoscopy on-air "experiment" had to be approved by NBC-TV honcho Jeff Zucker, who not only ran the entertainment network, but was already a colon cancer survivor who had been diagnosed at age 31.)

For the rest of us, especially perhaps men, talking about blood in our stools doesn't come so easily. That may be one reason why men are especially at risk...not a biological disadvantage as much as a cultural one: Middle-aged women, at least, have had decades of experience in talking with doctors about blood, menstrual blood, and how hormones and other bodily changes have affected their menses. This is New Stuff for the male of the species, even if and when we're led to the exam table by a smiling Couric and/or the other women who affect our lives and our health.

SURVIVORS' GUILT

Then, too, there is still more we (of both genders) don't talk about: After a war, a holocaust, a plane crash, you often hear people talk about "survivors' guilt." It's a known, studied phenomenon in psychology and psychiatry. Some years ago, I interviewed a Denver sales executive who quietly (for a sales guy, that is) had made a few million dollars in telemarketing and consulting. But instead of hanging all manner of corporate plaques hailing his accomplishments on his office walls, he had hung prominently, alongside his desk, a fading newspaper article that reported on a major, 1991 airplane crash in which 180 people had perished in the Midwest. This man, a thyroid cancer survivor, was supposed to be on that plane. He arrived so early, however, that he had qualified for a standby seat on a flight that left just one hour earlier.... Survivor's Guilt, perhaps? After all these years? Or does he continue to hang the harrowing clipping as simply a memento to being in the right place at the right time? He likes to think of this event, this near-death experience, as having more than a little to do with faith. The same goes for countless other cancer patients, I've found since my Stage III diagnosis a few years ago. Sometimes, whether we are ready or not, we're forced to "honor" the threats that have so impacted our lives. And ask the larger questions, the *largest* questions about life.

Having acknowledged this, though, the reason I still don't talk much about this possible guilt is that I still feel too damn hungry to survive. And from where I sit, despite mine and all the "NED" (No evidence of disease) anniversaries of my cancer brethren, I still believe I'm on shaky ground. I feel true empathy for my fellow cancer patients past and present, but the guilt, from a personal standpoint, I can't yet fathom. Perhaps it's because I'm unfeeling (despite appearances or what people who know me well have told me), but I don't honestly think that's the reason I'm not feeling the guilt pangs. Most things considered, the aversion to "celebrating" my survival-to-date probably has to do with a lingering sense of fear instead of finality. Plus, it has to do with a will to not carry others' burdens in ways I know I have in the past. Could it be possible, I wonder, that I won't be totally healed until I feel, acknowledge, even honor the haunting, hangdog emotion of survivor's guilt? If so, it's a stage that will bring up others' states of suffering. It's a stage, then, that I won't especially look forward to "achieving."

SURVIVORS' GRIT

For other patients, who've survived their first scare and yet still harbor cancer cells in their bodies, the up-down day-to-day existence is decidedly more trying than mine has been. For them and still others, it doesn't make emotional or physical sense to try to pretend the cancer's not there. (They don't have the "luxury" to ponder survivors' guilt, at least not yet.)

"I've had so much treatment and have been through two clinical trials," said Dubow "that the research [teams] kind of don't want me any more." With advanced disease, but as someone who outlived a handful of prognoses already, Lisa knew her long-term survival might be tied to continuing to think of herself as a patient...to keep searching for new therapies, new tacks to take when the standard ones played out. She was so steeped in colon cancer medicine fact she knew drug companies didn't necessarily want her on their drug-testing rosters. The reason is: As long as one keeps outliving the expected odds, the researchers following a case might wonder whether it's their particular drug that's responsible...for one's surprising longevity. "To have someone like me [survive] raises the question," Lisa said, matter-of-factly. "Is it their drugs that are working on me, or is it a combination of everything I've had *plus* their drugs? Those are some of the issues I've had."

Or, alternately, as Judy Webster, of Nebraska, says, "I know that life is so precious now, and that I've got to make every moment count.... I was told by my sister, 'Take one day at a time,' and I really think that we all should live that way. People say it...but what does that really mean? That you do have to stop, [slow down]? I'll look at the tree, and nature, and I'll see it in a different way, now. Appreciate it more. And I'll think about people who have died, and I'll think: 'I am here to enjoy these things, I'm going to enjoy them. Maybe this comes from being an artist, when I look at the sky, every night, I think about it. When I see the sunrise, I think about it...."

"I think it helps to talk about it," Judy adds, of the survivor's legacy. "And it has gotten better, people in general, I mean. They don't know what to say and they don't want to hurt your feelings. I didn't want to hurt my friends. Actually, what I wanted to do [when I found out about my cancer] was, I wanted to just go over there and hug my friend and hold her, and I couldn't do that either. Because it makes people feel funny. So you have to be 'up,' you have to have hope. And be strong for them because they don't want to see you weak.

"But," she concludes, " don't ever say, 'Oh, I know exactly how you feel.' I don't do that. I just say, 'I can relate to, somewhat, how you feel.' I don't [truly] know how you feel, but I can relate to it."

And Judy could probably relate quite well to what I felt, personally, a couple years ago, when I was still unsure of whether I'd make my two-year-all-clear; still trying to be "up" when so much uncertainty still hung, greasily, in the air....

FALSE ALARM?

"Waking on a cold morning, early winter," I wrote, "with a twinge astride my right testicle that ranges from groin to lower torso…uh-oh. Feels a little like a groin pull, but higher and connected to the dull, lingering pains I feel in my lower abdomen when I do push-ups or other ab work (not that I do a lot of 'ab-work.'). Surgery scar tissue, maybe, or worse? I make a note to ask about this pain at the next CT-scan checkup in two months…."

The months passed quickly, but not quickly enough…. "Driving south on Highway 36, heading out of the Boulder foothills and down to Denver," I added, "to see my oncologist, my reader of CT scans of abdomen, of pelvis, of chest, who checks for signs of angry, rogue cells. Passed the one-year mark okay, then the year-and-a-half…but for some reason the year and nine months has me jittery. Maybe it's because I'm a father now, maybe it's because I had that twinge…(though countless ex-cancer patients, I later learn, are forever mistaking twinges for recurrence).

"Here we go…and turns out I have no reason to worry. NED: No evidence of disease. No changes, apparently, from the study four months prior (love the way they call it a "study"). Dr. Cohn walks into the exam room and starts chatting with me about my recent stint in England. 'You likin' it over there?' Good news. If I had cancer signs, he wouldn't be talking tourism. 'You're healthy,' he says. I ask him to repeat this into my Sony micro cassette that I have placed on the chair next to me…(in case of bad news and my note-taking/thinking/reasoning collapsing). 'He's healthy!' Dr. Cohn says loudly to the Sony and thus to Paula, who will hear this tape at home after the baby wakes up. I smile as if I knew all along all would be okay (as if), and hop out to the car to call home. (You don't shout good news like this into a cell phone inside the Rocky Mountain Cancer Center…. Too many ill patients in attendance.)

"Now I'm back on the road, rolling north toward Highway 36 and home, feeling like I have just graduated from something big, singing along to a

Springsteen CD, pounding the steering wheel as a snare drum, or cymbal, as if I'm Tony Soprano in his Escalade.

> *These are better days, bay-buh /*
> *These are better days it's true /*
> *These are better days, bay-buh /*
> *There's better days shining through.*

SOLDIERING ON

Besides "Dr." Bruce Springsteen, one Canadian couple I talked with, two years after their Big Scare, helped me see quite clearly that there are better days ahead. They also nearly made me cry, when they talked about trying to put colon cancer behind them, maybe because I saw so much of Paula and myself mirrored back to me. Especially when Jayne, 38, talked about the new baby in the house, born just three months before Kenny's diagnosis in a Toronto hospital a few years ago. Jayne and Kenny, 41, and baby Amy, are out of the woods, you might say. But it wouldn't be quite right to call them gleeful. Least not yet....

"Sometimes I feel embarrassed by my 'notoriety,'" Jayne says. "You know, good wishes from long-unseen relatives and the like; you know you're being talked about and that it all sounds 'tragic.' And sometimes I feel amiss wondering what friends have noticed about me over the last couple of years. I wonder, though only fleetingly...if they think I am coming out of it okay.

"One of the 'little things,' and this is an understatement, that really almost irritates me, is the connection of a child and cancer being totally tragic to some people. You can tell in their tone. And for a quick (private) moment," Jayne says, "I want to *shriek*: "She gave us life–kept us *alive*–kept us together gave each day some shape!' But instead I find myself looking probably pious or something and say, quietly, 'but Amy was a joy; she kept us going.'

"[Still,] it is weird to hold all that joy and misery together in my mind," she says, speaking perhaps for both herself and her husband. "Sometimes I think it wasn't so bad (Kenny is a stoic, completely non-hysterical and from a medical family, unlike mine) and then I almost want to trip myself up and stab out, 'It was just awful,' while I remember Amy blowing raspberries at us at three months.... I also remember walking Amy around the old cemetery behind our house (it was near and I needed somewhere private to cry *loudly*–I couldn't do that at home and I couldn't go far because it still hurt to walk after Amy's birth–my pelvis was healing). I phoned a friend from work (of all people, and I called her before my parents and friends) and shrieked and cried from that cemetery.

"I also remember leaving Kenny in the city hospital, which did do a fantastic job, after all...the night before his surgery. And [I remember] seeing him full of fear, and going back down and out to the tarmac where my friends were wheeling Amy up and down. Two of my oldest friends and Ken's mom. I couldn't hold his hand all day post–op either, as I had Amy to deal with.

"Now I feel old and worried. We are so financially strapped—we have not and probably never will recover from 18 months-to-two years of no income at all. And I wonder whether Kenny's cancer will recur. And as you know, every twinge is something coming back. But on the other hand, which I always feel with this 'topic,' we are here, we are alive, Amy is a *joy* to us—true gorgeous joy and we're moving on. This year our garden might be good—so much died the summer Kenny was ill...and we've been busy since.

"Sometimes I think Kenny and I 'soldiered on' and pretended to each other, and kept the morale and chin up for so long that we became strangers to a degree, or were lacking some 'intimacy.' And even now—because we still cannot talk about cancer in the past tense—we are still in it and will be forever ensnared, I suppose. Even now we do not talk about those experiences that we *had* because our present and future is totally connected to all that."

This is what Jayne mostly said to me, shortly after I asked her to try and help me get a sense of how she and Kenny have put cancer "in its place." She didn't try to speak for him, in this instance. She was the spouse and caregiver (and new mom); not the patient. Turns out, though, that she didn't have to speak for him. Her words quite elegantly did the job for both. I'll not soon forget what she said about her family's bout with early, aggressive colon cancer. I'll not soon forget, either, the power of one comment she made to me: "This year our garden might be good."

Putting Fatigue in its Place

When your family and friends are calling (you know from Caller ID), it's tough, at first, to ignore the ring, to not answer the phone. But when you're recovering from colorectal cancer—or the chemo or radiation or surgery that's still fighting it—there are times where you know you've got to store your energy for just an hour or two of activity a day. And, cancer patients know too well, talking on the phone (about your body and disease) constitutes activity. Fatigue, we know, is no small matter.

Not long ago, medical researchers found that cancer-related fatigue is more important than they had previously believed. In studies at H. Lee Moffitt Cancer Center, Tampa, Florida, Dr. Paul Jacobsen and colleagues tried treating fatigue with new substances (i.e., EPO, for anemia-like conditions) and medicines, instead of merely relying on talk therapy...and the passage of time. They were pleasantly, and repeatedly surprised.

"Fatigue is exacerbated by depression, emotional distress and stress," says Dr. Jacobsen. "And cancer patients experience high levels of stress and distress, especially during treatment." Which only, he adds, exacerbates their fatigue. Patients won't always mention their fatigue because they expect it, or feel they should just accept it—the "cancer" part of healing seems more important to discuss.

"It's the silent symptom," Jacobsen adds, "because patients don't realize they are suffering a symptom." Until now, and possibly for months past the last treatment, patients and caregivers haven't realized how many ways there are available to fight fatigue, and to help put this side-effect behind them.

For more info on the studies, or related treatment, contact:
National Colorectal Cancer Research Alliance/ EIF: 1-800- 872- 3000; www.nccra.org; or H. Lee Moffitt Cancer Center, Paul Jacobsen, Ph.D., 813-979-7295.

CHAPTER 3

Friends and Family: The Other Survivors

"It's not fair." Course it's not. Yet when I say I thought that thought during the worst stages of my treatment, I wasn't thinking only about sad-sack me. It was Paula I was thinking about, who, yes, vowed to care for me "in sickness," but who, like me, never thought the need would arise so soon. This was our sixth year of marriage; not our twenty-sixth, nor forty-sixth. Not fair.

For far too long Paula ran my life; she ran my bath. She ran my treatment schedules; she cooked, blended, chopped, shopped and looked for the light through all the dark. She took the tough phone calls; she shuttled me to-and-fro the hospital wards and blood-draw rooms that smelled, faintly, of disinfectant. Like a trainer guiding a gimpy halfback to the sidelines, she'd sling her arm around me when I was wob-

> " As someone who has spent his entire adult life dealing with cancer in a clinical setting, I've found the true miracles of cancer rarely take the form of drugs, potions, or herbs. More often than not, the true miracles take place in the minds, hearts, and spirits of patients and their families. "
>
> – Jeremy Geffen, M.D., and author, *The Journey Through Cancer*

bly from fatigue, and lead me down the stairs to the sunken radiation rooms. Other times at home, she played bouncer—keeping a few energy-sapping souls from getting too-too near to us, when it all seemed too exhausting. Post-op, sleeping overnight in my room, she handled my urgent food-drink-bedpan needs when the metal staples in my stomach were fresh—and when a man in my condition needed the toughest advocate he could find. When I got a little better, she was my lover again, though we were a hundred times more careful than we'd ever been.

Through the worst of it, Paula won the big battles on my behalf, as my wife/partner/friend. And yet there was so little I could do, in that state, for her in return. I mouthed thank-yous; I told her that I loved her. Inside I vowed to try with everything I had to get stronger, to get better. For her *and* for me. Then, after a few hopeful scans and blood-test check-ups, once I started to believe I might actually be around a few years, I began to think about her circumstances: My wife deserved better. Still does. "It's not fair."

ME, CANCER, AND GEOFF

One of the things I couldn't get from my wife, from Day One of diagnosis through Year Three follow-up, was black humor. Healing black humor. That was most often delivered by my best friend, for whom life wasn't fair either—ever since his mother died of cancer when he was 13. If Paula was my Rock, Geoff was my hard place.

Calling in from Chicago, while I'm still in shock-awe about a malignant tumor in my body, he says, "I got an idea. You can do a book; call it: *Me, Cancer, and Geoff.* Instead of a book about how you and your wife got through this together, it'll be a buddy book about how I helped you kick cancer. I'll be calling you every day; people aren't expecting that." Pause.

"You're sick," I say.

"I know," he says. "But I gotta ask you: Does this mean I'll have to do one of those Run-Walk things with you in five years?"

(Addendum: In fall, 2004, I invited Geoff, my friend for 33 years, to accompany me in the 5K, fund-raising "Snoopy Walks to End Colon Cancer," activists' event in Washington, D.C., in honor of "Peanuts" creator Charles M. Schulz, who died of colon cancer in 2000. Half expected Geoff to show up last-minute, clad in a zig-zag Charlie Brown sweater.)

GO TEAM (Part I)

As anyone who's fought cancer knows, it's an understatement to say it helps to have help. Not just for physical demands, but for the longer-term, psychological ones as well. You're not alone in your hurt. We know that: Been there, felt that. We also *think* we know that because so much needs to be done, the sooner the patient can get back to "normal," the better.... But recovery isn't that simple. Especially when those closest to you have assumed multiple, integral roles in your daily life. At one point I remembered thinking, "How do I show I'm not so damn dependent?"

One of the first things I did, even before my surgery when I could neither handle stairs nor walk two blocks outside by myself, was push-ups. Not bolt-straight, military "Drop down and Gimme Fifty!" push-ups, but 10-to-20 pseudo-push-ups. "Girly" push-ups, Gov. Schwarzenegger might call 'em. I'd stand at the foot of the bed, or at the sturdy bathroom sink, take a step back, and do a dozen or more lean-to exercises, lowering, then slowly raising, my body from a measly, 60- or 75-degree angle back up to 90.

I wasn't going after biceps at this point: I was aiming for minimal maintenance of what muscle I had left. Also, I was trying to show my wife—my teammate—that each and every night, whether it actually helped or not, I would and could do something for myself.... Wanted her to see I had some strength left; wanted her to see I was determined to be more of a man again. I wanted her to know that she wasn't in this—no matter how she might have felt—alone.

Months later, when I was much, much stronger (but still wondering whether I was carrying half our marriage's "load"), I came across an apt passage from author Jeremy Geffen, M.D., an oncologist who wrote *The Journey Through Cancer*: "Remember that your spouse and family cannot meet all of your emotional needs. It is unfair and unwise to ask them to do so. You can help yourself, and them, by finding other places for support."

Note to self: Is now the time for me finally to knock on the door of the Colorado colon cancer support group's local chapter? Do they do push-ups in there?

DO THE MATH

Instead of doing push-ups, Shari Rogoff, 38, of Englewood, New Jersey, did the math. After caring for both her mother, who died of uterine cancer in 1999, and her father, who died of colon cancer in 2001at age 62, it came time for her to make a survivor's plan, rather early in life: "What's the best way for me to avoid getting cancer?" she asked. She admired greatly her dad's spirit and fight through then advanced stages of his disease; the fact that he'd even voted for taking powerful, radiation treatments near the end of his life. He did so, in hopes that "if I hang on, I might make it to the experimental trial of that ImClone." Genetically-speaking, she didn't much like the DNA she'd been dealt.

"I was told," she says, "not to worry about a colonoscopy till I was 49," she says. "That's 10 years down the road. It'd be the age at which my dad's cancer was diagnosed. But I told my doctor that's not good enough. Because if you do the math, and believe me, I did it, you'll figure that colon cancer cells can develop and hide in polyps for years before they're diagnosed. So I subtracted another 10 from my dad's age and made an appointment for a colonoscopy. I was 38. Sure enough, the doctor woke me from the twilight drugs and said, 'We found three polyps and took them out.' The next week, when the pathology report came back, my doctor called me and told me they were the kind that turn into cancer. I got lucky, and, literally, saved my ass.

"I was supposed to come back and get another colonoscopy in three years, but I wasn't satisfied with that. So the doctor recommended I come back for a repeat colonoscopy in two. I said, 'What would you do if I came back in one year for a follow-up?' He said, 'I'd give you a Valium and send you home.' But if I hadn't done the math," Rogoff says, "I would definitely have had colon cancer."

GO TEAM (Part II)

At some of my worst times, physically, I was also blessed to have a seamless stream of close family members, flying to see me in San Francisco, all from Chicago. They came, one-at-a-time at pre-arranged times and weeks (to spread the total visit time) to help with my care; Mom, Dad, sister Beth (whose husband Howard initiated Sabbath prayers for me every Saturday, for months on the homefront). Out of my earshot they'd worked it all out with Paula: the details of who was coming when. I had no clue. But I knew I was never... alone. During these stretches I felt comforted, maybe a little wigged out, but as close to back-in-the-womb as a middle-aged, seriously diseased man could climb. With intimate, selfless support like this, I remember thinking, Could I actually consider myself "lucky?"

TAG TEAM

No way did Helen Lyman, at age 68, consider herself lucky during her colon cancer fight. For starters, she received a Stage IV diagnosis; one that, at first, looked rather grim. "I had a lot of pain in the appendix; cancer was found; they took it out," she says, matter-of-factly. "I was fine. Then I [got] diverticulitis and was misdiagnosed: They gave me pain meds and I went on to China, where I was teaching for the State Department. The pain persisted, until they did a scope, and surgery and chemo...." Worse news followed, but she rebounded. "I'm not supposed to be around," she says, again matter-of-factly.

"Obviously, it's always a shock when you get the diagnosis," says her husband, Princeton Lyman, a State Department veteran and former U.S. ambassador to Nigeria and South Africa. "And Helen's attitude was absolute determination to fight the disease. But you want to share that....

"Helen didn't want to be alone in the hospital," says Princeton, "because she was alone when she was told she had only a 15 percent chance of recovery. [What happened was] the oncologist had made his rounds late at night; and I was working and couldn't be there."

Adds the ambassador: "I don't listen to those statistics any longer— because that was devastating for us." The statistics said Helen should have died some years ago. These days, he says of his wife, "You don't tell someone how to feel. Helen got angry for a while, at the pain.... So sometimes I 'let her' feel discouraged. It's alright to let someone be a little angry."

A KEY DE-STRESSOR

Once the shock and anger fades, a patient's support team tends to get... analytical. Oftentimes the focus turns to: "Who is to blame for this disaster?" And, in many cases, rightly so. But over the long-term, over years of hoped-for survival, the patient and caregivers benefit more when they try to replace anger, negative energy or stress with more positive emotions. Admittedly, this is easier said, and written, than done. Especially with so many still-unknown links between the mind and body.

While stress is known to negatively affect our health in various ways, can it cause cancer? Can we blame it? "This is the era of stress causing everything in the world. It's very unfortunate," says Barrie Cassileth, Ph.D., director of Memorial Sloan-Kettering Cancer Center's integrative medicine unit in New York City and author of *Alternative Medicine Handbook: The Complete Reference Guide to Alternative and Complementary Therapies.* "There certainly is a mind-body link, but I don't think the mind causes cancer and I don't think the mind can cure it."

From this point on, if you believe Cassileth's take (and after interviewing her, I became a disciple) it becomes clear that stress-management—through music, DVDs, massage, tears or quiet talks—can be a worthy goal of patients, friends and family. Dealing with stress is no longer just a "to-do" to cross off one's list after yoga class. After all, as long as it's (undeniably) here, your goal and that of your caregiver(s) shifts a bit.

According to Cassileth, reactions to major health stresses tend to cause some fairly predictable, or automatic, behaviors.

Knowing now what to expect may help navigate them in the future:

- temporary denial
- connecting with loved ones
- imposing structure or order in a new setting or life phase
- connecting spiritually through prayer or meditation
- reaching out to others in need

FEELINGS...

Sometimes it's just plain tough to reach out, on either side of the invisible wall that surrounds each newly diagnosed patient. That was how Judy Webster, then 56, of Omaha, Nebraska, felt (see pg. 67), when she literally tried to reach over to some folks she thought would understand her needs to re-connect, soon after her new diagnosis of colorectal cancer. "I didn't want to hurt my friends, who didn't know what to say...or how to act," Webster says.

"What I wanted to do was just go over there and hug my friend and hold her, and you couldn't do that either, because it makes people feel funny. So you have to be 'up'; you have to have hope and be strong for them. Because they don't want to see you weak. Just try to be strong for them, I guess." Which is one way to de-stress the circumstances, albeit not an easy way.

HOME ALONE

The patient from Wilmington, Sara-Jo Matthys, 46, didn't want me to take this the wrong way. During her first bout with breast cancer, in her early 40s, she was alone, but not totally alone. For we both knew, as cancer survivors who shared a mutual friend, that her marriage ended in divorce in the early 1990s, long before her diagnosis. "I got married way too young," she said. "I had just graduated college, at 22. He was an older guy, a photographer, and I got swept along."

By the time she was diagnosed and treated for breast cancer, however, she was 43 years old, and barely into a relationship. So when it came time to deal with the scare of her life, she had no husband or life partner to help her through the ordeal. "I did have a boyfriend at the time," she says. "He bailed out. He was there during the diagnosis, but left after a couple months. He told me 'I'm just really not a good caretaker.' So I guess he wasn't the man for me for whatever reason.

"Around that time, I remember thinking...'Am I gonna lose my breast? My hair? My boyfriend? Is he gonna care? Or be grossed out?' I became my sole support."

For most of her treatment, Sara-Jo was alone. She worked at her home-based consulting business; she often dragged herself to all manner of doctor and hospital appointments. Aging, infirm, parents, just one out-of-town sibling…two more reasons her friends were her last leg of support. (And her saving grace, she told me later.) But one weekend early in her treatment, a friend drove nine hours to spend two weeks with her and keep her company through a rough patch.

"I was crying for the entire weekend right after surgery," says Matthys. "I had problems with my [post-surgical] drains. My friend came to say things like: 'You're sooo negative. You've got to stop thinking about this stuff 24/7.'

"How could I not think that way? I realized then-and-there I didn't want to inflict this on someone else. If I wanted to cry myself to sleep, which I did a lot, then having someone sitting in the other room, freaking out, wasn't going to help me. There was nothing she could do for me. Unlike your family, I didn't feel I could be—or let her be—unconditional in our roles. I came to realize I didn't want to burden her. When it came time for me to get injections of Neupogen for 10 days straight, after treatment, I learned how to inject myself with a hypodermic syringe. And I know…it would have been different with a husband or boyfriend."

CHEMO BY THE BAY

Thing about cancer is, nobody wants to be there: Not the patient; not his wife or family; not even his docs, sometimes, if we're all telling the truth here. And usually not his friends. They all have families and careers and wives or exes—and other friends, too. So it was surprising to me, amazing actually, when I realized maybe eight weeks into my ordeal, that a dozen, maybe even more, of my friends, were reaching out to me: physically, emotionally, prayerfully, financially, medically, even comically.

This was powerful stuff, to a midlife patient in crisis. Could relationships such as this, I wondered at times, actually help the chemo and radiation do its stuff? At one point I looked back and wrote:

"Easing into a leatherette La-Z-Boy in the UCSF infusion center, waiting for my blood work and for two friends to come by. (Farley's a San Fran local; Pete'll fly in from Denver for a few hours.) Suddenly I hear Paula say, 'Oh, my God, there's Brandy!'—meaning my grade-school friend who's joined by my high-school bud Jerry, which means we're having a surprise San Francisco-chemo-by-the-Bay party, only half of which I was expecting....

Can't believe these guys pulled this one off—that with four wives and thirteen kids among them, they were able to shuck their schedules, blow off clients, and see if they couldn't give me some old-style, are-we-ever-gonna-grow-up, ball-busting support. On a day I might not feel much like partying.

For the occasion, Farley rents a 1450cc Harley (which Brandy falls off of while stopped at a stoplight); Pete raids the free (!) graham-crackers-and-apple-juice "for patients only" pantry; and Jerry makes gross jokes about the rubber gloves he doesn't seem to want to take off.... I'm back in high school again, laughing my head off with old friends...till the drugs make me weak and the airport calls the boys home.

Caregiver Tips: What to Say
...or Not to Say

When you get news that cancer has hit someone close to home or work, here are some patient-tested guidelines to help keep the "care" in caregiver:

WHAT TO SAY:

- Useful information is welcome, but random stories of other colon cancer patients with sad—or happy—endings are not.
- Instead of: "Call me if there's anything I can do," let the patient know you'll be bringing something by. And when. For even the most widely used, genuine, offer has a glitch: A family in cancer crisis has no time to dole out chores. Get a solid idea for a good deed and simply do it.
- "I / we love you." (Can't hear that one enough.)
- "You don't need to call/write/email back." Patients appreciate being let off the hook.
- "We've added you to our prayer circle." (Can't hear this one enough.)
- "I / we love you." (Told you we patients can't hear that one enough.)

WHAT NOT TO SAY:

- Before you ask a patient whether their type of cancer "runs in the family," you might first ask yourself: "I wonder how many times this question's been asked." Then consider: Even if it does run in the family, how exactly will this answer help the newly-diagnosed patient feel or get better? (On the flip side, if there is no hereditary/genetic link, might this imply that the cancer patients did something to "cause" their cancer to develop?)
- If you say something from the *faux pas* file, apologize. But cancer patients get to say anything they want.
- Never tell a balding man who's losing his few survivors to chemo, "Well, there wasn't much there, anyway."
- "I know how you feel." You can't.

What to Do...or Not to Do

WHAT TO DO:

- You have a license to be angry. Feel free to use it...occasionally.
- Laughter is healing; silly joke gifts are not.
- Listen carefully; take notes for the patient and keep your comments simple. A gleam of acknowledgment goes a long way. A good go-to: "Just wanted to let you know that I'm thinking about you and praying for you."
- Acknowledge or grieve for what you've lost; give yourself/yourselves permission to forge ahead with new plans and dreams.
- Kiss a receptionist: Well, not literally. But when acting as advocate for a family member or friend, there's more to the role than coordinating docs, medicines, meals and insurance. That's why it pays, literally, to always ask—and jot down— the name(s) of those who help you along the way. The best receptionists and office-assistants can save a cancer patient time, money and discomfort. (They can also magically move your chart or results in front of a doctor's eyes much more quickly if they get to know you—and like you.) So spend the extra minute or two—no need to be cloying—each visit and try to wrangle the front-office worker onto your team.

WHAT NOT TO DO:

- Don't give unsolicited self-help books, at first. The last thing a new cancer patient needs is to feel guilty about the stack of unread "How to Get Betters" beside the bed.
- Don't tell them how to feel. They may not want to play the 'glad' game, and instead might want to indulge in maudlin humor. It's their call.
- Don't be a drain. Keep those random horror stories, gloomy statistics, far, far away.
- Don't ignore your own needs. When was the last time you took a walk? Or spent quality time with...yourself? Don't feel guilty about caring for yourself as well as the patient.
- Don't be afraid to contact a support group or therapist if you sense a shift from fatigue to despair or depression.

Caregiver Solutions

Today, with about 10 million cancer survivors living in the U.S., the field of caregiving has moved beyond booming...to sprawling. Here are a few time-tested and respected places to find support for caregivers when you're feeling, at times, as if you've got nothing left to give:

- The National Coalition for Cancer Survivorship: the original grassroots advocacy and survival organization.
www.canceradvocacy.org 877-622-7937

- National Family Caregivers Association
www.nfcacares.org 301-942-6430

- Cancer Recovery Foundation of America: includes therapy-guided treatment sources and spiritual advice.
www.cancerrecovery.org 800-238-6479

- *Today's Caregiver* magazine: **www.caregiver.com 800-829-2734**

CHAPTER 4

Medical Matters: New Treatments, Long-Life Strategies

It's no accident that one of the world's most prestigious colon cancer treatment sites looks, from the bustling streetscape of York Avenue in New York City, much like the NBC *Today* show studio in Rockefeller Center. The broad windows, the oversize plasma screens visible from the sidewalk, the digital electronica, the scrolling zippered lines of medical info, steadily pulsing, drawing you closer. It's all there, except maybe Matt Lauer.

For on March 30, 2004, the celebrated day The Jay Monahan Center for Gastrointestinal Health opened on campus at New York Presbyterian Hospital/Weill Cornell Medical Center, the hot lights of television newsfolk flicked on and filming began—as if to say: "Colon cancers of the

" We have too many agents; we don't know how to mix them together in the right order. But that's a luxury to have, because five years ago we didn't have much. "

– Louis Fehrenbacher, M.D., medical oncologist with Kaiser Permanente, in *The New York Times*, Feb. 27, 2004 future, we're ready to beat you now." First came the doctors, explaining how this new "all-in-one" treatment center will seek to be a model of world-class colorectal cancer care and prevention. Next came NBC-TV's Katie Couric, introduced to (and cheered by) a crowd of more than 200 media, medical and donor types. "Most importantly," she said of the large staff drawn to work at the new center named for her late husband, "they *get* it—they know how to help patients during one of the worst possible experiences of their lives."

This was today, not on NBC.

THE CELEBRITY PRESCRIPTION

Inside a temporary white tent and flanked by colon cancer bigwigs, Couric & Co. welcomed dozens of press and scores of supporters to the near-glitzy, ground-floor facility designed with families in mind. "There's no (traditional) waiting room," said Mark Bennett Pochapin, M.D. director of the Center, while guiding a tour through the facility. "...[Not] only do patients receive the cutting-edge in gastrointestinal cancer prevention and treatment, they do so in a way that is compassionate. You see, this looks more like a living room." Indeed, patients are as likely to see an early *Harry Potter* DVD playing on the television as they are a documentary-style video on colonoscopy (though that's available, too, for the asking.) The home-like environment was in part Couric's idea, along with input from her hospital-based colleagues and those from the Los Angeles-based Entertainment Industry Foundation (EIF), of which she is an unusually active member. Much of the funding to build the Center flowed in following the efforts of Couric and the EIF Broadway-meets-Hollywood fundraisers that brought in millions of dollars in donations.

"How do you find the best treatment? What is the best treatment? Are clinical trials available?... What complementary therapies might boost your chances for success?" asked Couric of the crowd. "What should you be eating? How do you deal with the side effects of treatment? How do you deal, *period?*" As she spoke, Couric and her sister-in-law, Clare Myers, Jay Monahan's sister, had tears in their eyes: a heartfelt private-public moment. In fact, since 1998, Couric and her family have dealt with the loss of her husband, from advanced colon cancer, with uncommon grace and a model, give-back attitude. Even after moving to CBS News in 2006, Couric has kept colon cancer activism alive on multiple fronts.

One of the first things Couric did to help alter the nature of colon cancer treatment was to point out the significance of early detection. For the bold statistic still stands: Some 90 percent of colorectal cancer cases can be cured outright if the disease is caught early, in Stage I of the four (IV) main stages of cancer development. Instead of merely advising her morning show viewers to get a colonoscopy to find polyps or early-stage disease, she decided to have her own colonoscopy filmed—and broadcast—to more than five million people in March 2000. Turned out her insides were pink, healthy (she smiled for the camera, though clearly sedated). It also turned out that this bold act led to a massive and unprecedented increase across America among younger men and women getting screened for colon cancer symptoms for the first time. Docs at the University of Michigan dubbed this national, year-2000-era increase in the numbers of patients screened, "The Couric Effect."

THE PATIENT'S EDGE (Part I)

Jon Henderson, of Boulder, Colorado, was a guitar-playing broadcaster who, like Couric, knew a bit about like cancer advocacy himself. Following his diagnosis of Stage IV colon cancer in 1999, I eventually met Jon via an oncologist who treated us both. At first glance, Jon, at 48, a lean, sweaty guy doing barbell curls in the far corner of the gym with a trainer, didn't look much to me like a colon cancer advocate. Nor did Henderson look like someone who also had spent 45 days in a surgery-induced coma. Then again, Henderson, an eight-year Stage IV colon cancer survivor, delighted in knocking down stereotypes about what middle-aged survivors are supposed to look like—and how they're supposed to feel. At second glance, face-to-face with Henderson in the gym, I couldn't help but notice the portable oxygen tank at his side, with nostril tubes snaking up and clipped into place. That wasn't from the colon can-cer—well, not exactly. It was from surgery on metastatic tumors in his lungs that led them to shut down, a condition known as adult respiratory distress syn-drome that put him into a prolonged unconsciousness. Post-op, if he didn't push himself like this in the gym, chances are he wouldn't need the oxygen feed, said Jon's trainer Kevin Schoeninger. Yet he was determined to get stronger, in more ways than one. "Once people know you have it—can-cer—they look at you a whole different way," Henderson said. "It's the 'dead-man-walking' look. But once you get out there, you can educate friends and family. In my case, we've been looking at this as treating a chronic [as opposed to fatal] disease for almost eight years. That makes it a little more acceptable, and people feel better about it when they're around you."

THE PATIENT'S EDGE (PART II)

At this point of Jon's story a few things should be said: First, an average Stage IV colon cancer patient, with a similar diagnosis 15 or 20 years ago, wouldn't have been alive for me to interview eight years later. Nor would that patient have been pumping iron in a modern gym. Today we can now expect many Stage IVs, as Jon said, to be treated as those who have a "chronic" disease. That doesn't belittle the severity of the diagnoses. (Indeed, Henderson died in early 2008; his charity-driven documentary/CD, Big C, is stocked at Rocky Mountain Cancer Centers Foundation, Denver, 303-930-7822 or: www.rmccf.org)

Instead, these new patient outlooks offer a new, more personalized view of treating some advanced cancer cases with various advanced, FDA-approved and combined cancer medicines. From 5-FU to FOLFOX and FOLFIRI, to new radiation schemes and bio-chemo-cocktails that include Avastin, Eloxatin, Erbitux and Vectibix, all manner of Stage III and IV survivors have an entirely different menu from which to choose than what was presented to me, circa 2001. In short the field of advanced cancer treatment has become at once more hopeful and more complex.

CEA: A SURVIVOR'S SURVEILLANCE TEST

It's not infallible and it is, at times, open to misinterpretation. But for colorectal cancer patients interested in monitoring the likelihood of tumor recurrence, the CEA (carcinoembryonic antigen) blood test is worth getting to know. At levels of 1.0- to 3.0 ng/ml, CEA is typically termed normal. At levels in the 40s and 50s ng/ml, CEA can be considered extremely high. (Yet still, not totally conclusive for recurrence, as CEA levels may also become elevated due to inflammatory bowel disease, such as colitis; or even liver disease.) With the newer courses of chemo and biologic drugs, docs often have seen—and are now used to seeing—readings that start out near 50 drop down into the 20s ng/ml after initial therapy. Then too, smokers' CEA results may also run higher than average, without pointing to cancer recurrence."

A DOC SPEAKS: SURGERY

Not long after Henderson joined an experimental study that involved some of the first biologics-paired-with-chemo drugs, Daniel Haller, M.D., of Abramson Cancer Center at the University of Pennsylvania, was asked to help educate countless patients, during an online seminar about options available to the colon cancer community. As every case is unique, how does a patient find perspective?

"What happens if you get [colon cancer]," he said, "well, you're going to meet up with a surgeon because in most cases, the treatment is going to be surgical. Right now the only people considered for a colostomy are people with [rare conditions or] tumors on the last inch or two of the rectum. In the past, many people were afraid to get a colonoscopy because they feared colostomy, but very few people need that. Most people simply need the section of their intestine removed [resection, it's called] where there is the tumor. Very simple."

SURGICAL STRIKE: A PATIENT RECONSIDERS

"Simple?" As author of this book and an ex-patient who left his colon and rectum in the operating room some years ago (I was one of the unfortunate 15 percent who faced colostomy-type surgery, due to both the site and Stage III of my cancer, plus years of intermittent ulcerative colitis when I was younger), simple is not a word I would use to describe any type of surgery of this sort. With all due respect to Doc Haller, this is how I described my "Opening Day," in my journal, soon after I received it:

"Three weeks ago...a couple of doctors I knew, and eight of whom I didn't, gathered in the OR of Moffitt Hospital at UCSF to put me under, take me apart, and put me back together. They gathered that Tuesday in April to try to make me a Stage III patient who used to have cancer. They gathered to take on a disease that grew for years by division—cell division—and yet the success of their surgery would hinge on collaboration.

"There would be no room for error, really. A strike in baseball—'Steeeee-riiiike!!!' —means a pitcher's hit his catcher's target. A successful surgical strike in cancer-speak means They Got It All, with 'clear margins'." Turns out the sonsagun done committed a successful surgical strike, oncologically speaking. Those Sonsagun surgeons, Dr. Mark Lane Welton and Dr. Peter Carroll, came strutting down the hall after eight hours of tough surgery on my body and my malignancy; sonsagun came down the hall in their surgical blues, smiling like they'd done roped the biggest mean-ass steer at the state fair ro-*de*-o. I'd tip my ten-gallon to 'em, but I'm still unconscious, waiting to wake up in the recovery room and hear Paula repeat what the doctors told me but I did not hear: that I am cancer-free. For now at least; hopefully till the day I die. Of other causes. Sonsaguns hit the mitt."

Simple?

A DOC SPEAKS: SURGERY AND STAGING

"When we remove the tumor or the polyp that contains the tumor," Haller goes on to say, "that's when we think about staging. 'What is my stage?' patients want to know. It's really quite simple: the reason we care is that the stage relates to prognosis…. We hope we find the tumor residing *inside* the lining of the colon, the inner part. It starts on the inner part and it grows outward, and as it grows outwardly through the colon, it can get into the wall, the muscular wall of the colon, from which it can grow through the wall." Stage I is, as most survivors' know, the least invasive; the best-case scenario (that is, besides hearing, "Your polyps were benign.").

Increasingly, depending on the stage and severity of one's cancer, doctors like Haller are making surgical decisions they didn't face five or 10 years ago. Such as: Should they operate on this patient laparoscopically (using pinpoint "keyhole" surgery and image-guided tools and miniature cutting blades), or traditionally (meaning a wider/larger, longer incision, often called "open" surgery)? The debates about which technique is "better" for colon tumors won't be solved right away, but evidence is mounting that the former has its advantages. As experts have seen in the fields of knee and hernia surgery…once doctors complete a "learning" period, laparoscopic surgery in most fields, performed well, can help patients recover more quickly and leave the hospital sooner, often with no compromise in terms of safety or long-term prognosis.

In fact, in cases of rectal (but not colon) cancer, a new procedure known as TME—total mesorectal excision—has come to be seen as both revolutionary and "nerve-sparing," over the past decade. It enables cancer surgeons to remove more diseased, and potentially diseased tissue than was possible before TME entered the field…but at the same time saving countless patients' sexual and urinary function (i.e. nerves) that formerly might have been nicked, cut or lost during rectal excisions of the past. While not all surgeons have yet practiced this tricky but patient-friendly cancer surgery dozens of times (luckily for me, mine did), according to Mark Lane Welton, M.D., colorectal surgeon and associate professor at Stanford University's medical school, those who have are able to offer rectal cancer patients an improved lifestyle, better sexual function, and improved chance of cure.

Haller continues: "If the tumor goes through the wall, in some patients, microscopic cells could have already gotten into the circulation through the lymph nodes and lymph stream or the bloodstream—and the vast percentage of those patients, 80 percent, are cured by surgery. But now we have a situation where 15-to-20 percent of the patients will have cells that will grow and be found within five years after surgery." This is how recurrence occurs…and Haller explains that if it involves the lymph system, it is more widespread. "We call it Stage III, although even in this scenario, surgeons cure patients. And medical oncologists and radiologists can increase the cure rate, too…" among those patients who've had 'positive' nodes [those that contained cancer cells when studied in the lab after surgery]. "In that case," Dr. Haller concludes, "having one node is better than 10."

THE PATIENT'S EDGE (Part III)

Fred Holper, 48, a Stage IV patient/advocate from New Jersey whom I talked with in 2004 and 2006, had positive nodes. That was the first step of advanced colon cancer that led to discovery of tumors in his liver, his METS. So, following his first six-week cycle of chemotherapy, he explained, "They gave me a drug that was called an antiangiogenesis drug, or 'Veg-Ef for short, or they called it by its generic name [bevacizumab]. And about a year ago [in 2003] we finally got a name attached about it, Avastin. I remember saying: 'Am I gonna live long enough to see the FDA approve this?' So last year, it was two years since I was diagnosed. In the beginning, I said, this stuff is wiping me out…but I've been on it two years." In fact, without this drug, some doctors believe Holper wouldn't have lived much longer than one year; he ultimately lived five years beyond his diagnosis.

"After the first six weeks, I go for my next CAT scan," Holper told me in an interview, "and I see 'them' again on the screen. I say to my doc: 'The tumors LOOK smaller.' Now, I don't have calipers with me, or anything: But here I am, looking at them with a picture of what they used to look like, in my mind.... 'They certainly don't look bigger,' is what I'm thinking. Three days later I saw [my doc again] at the beginning of my next chemo cycle.... And now he has his calipers: Turns out the tumors are about 50 percent smaller. I say, 'That's good, isn't it?' He said, 'Wow, that's incredible!'"

The associated lab work looked good, according to his doctor. Patient Holper's CEA (or carcinoma-embryonic antigen level) went from a reading of 44, which was skyscraper-high at time of surgery, down to 24 after the first cycle of chemo and Avastin; an encouraging sign. After the second six-week cycle, the CEA dropped way down to 3, which was exciting to both Holper and his medical team. Because when it comes to reading CEA blood tests, a measure of 1-to-3 is considered normal (smokers' results may run a bit higher). "My mother's CEA was about a 3, but when she [her cancer] metastasized she shot way up. When mine dropped to 3, I went, 'Hey, that's good. I'll take that.'" When he punched out that result, Holper's voice carried more than mere hints of his Central Jersey, cum-Tony-Soprano-accent.

SURVIVORS' CHEMO 101

Somewhere between those who need(ed) no chemo and have an extremely good prognosis, and those who face the grueling course of chemotherapy that Holper had to take, is a place I know pretty well. When diagnosed with my Stage III disease, I was too ill to bypass chemo, but not ready for immediate surgery. And I also wasn't ready (or my tumor hadn't "advanced" enough) for the yet-unproven Big Gun drugs as there were saftey concerns. So I was placed on a course of chemotherapy that included two basic drugs: 5-FU, or flouroracil, and leucovorin, which have worked well together in fighting colorectal cancer since the 1960s. However, because of the size and particular location of my tumor, my docs at University of California-San Francisco opted to infuse me with a six-week, low-dose course of the drugs *before* my surgery. They operated to insert a catheter into my chest; then fitted me with a portable pump and a waist-pack, that together would keep the drugs flowing into my body pretty much nonstop. (I slept with the pack under my pillow. Sweet frickin' dreams....)

The goal: to shrink the tumor in and around the rectum enough in 12 weeks time, so that the surgeons could, (A) remove it completely; (B) be able to verify a "clear margin" of cancer-free tissue around the site; and (C) leave-my-prostate-gland-the-heck-alone. If the prostate were "involved," my prognosis (and sex life) would forever be much worse. Not all colon cancer tumors crowd the prostate, of course...former President Ronald Reagan's didn't in the 1980s; nor did ex-major league ballplayer Eric Davis's in the 1990s, neither did Sharon Osbourne's, of Ozzy-the-rock-star and television fame, in the early 2000s (that's right, women have no prostate gland, but fortunately her colon cancer hadn't invaded her ovaries).

The toughest part of this "neo-adjuvant" (pre-surgical) therapy, at the time and in retrospect, was that I had to decide it made more sense to leave the tumor in my body for a few (3) months, instead of voting for an operation right away. I was choosing to live with "living" cancer longer than I had to, in hopes of—if the treatment, radiation and surgery all clicked—having complete remission and ultimately, a cure. That is how much I came to trust my team at UCSF. I chose to keep cancer—and play the oncological odds.

DOCSPEAK 101: THE NEW CHEMO AND BIO-THERAPY DRUGS

A few years later, about 3 years after my surgery, as it happens, I had a chance to interview one of my doctors, Alan Venook, M.D., medical oncologist and a nationally-known, leading researcher at UCSF. While he was pleased to learn I was in remission—and once again running and mountain biking, he also took some time to put chemo for patients and other survivors into better perspective. Of course we should all be thrilled with the recent approval of new colorectal cancer drugs like Avastin and Erbitux, Venook said. Yet he felt compelled to point out that the new drugs don't work for everybody... and that they aren't yet in wide use for Stage III ex-patients like myself, or Stage I or II, either. Those experiments (and ultimately wider approval from the Food and Drug Administration [FDA]) will take maybe a decade to filter down into the mainstream.

"Cancers are deceitful diseases and they really have figured out how to resist therapies by developing multiple pathways and multiple physiologic mechanisms to escape from inhibition," Venook says. "I think it's incredibly exciting, but I think truly at the end of the day...the real trick, the challenge in research is going to be not to treat 100 patients to help the 10." What he means is: Wouldn't we be better off pre-selecting patients, before each chemo course, who are the most likely to actually benefit from each particular medicine?

Of course we would, but we aren't there yet: patients, survivors, or 'med-oncs' like Venook. The good news, the encouraging news, is that there are now a host of truly good possibilities for recurrent or advanced colon cancer patients to try. From surgery to single-courses of chemo to newer combinations like FOLFOX (a mix of 5-FU, leucovorin and oxaliplatin) and more. But there still will be a good number of failures. We are, you might say, at a place in medicine akin to where HIV/AIDS patients were in the late 1980s and early 1990s: when drugs were few and AZT was still

the best hope, medically, for extending the lives of AIDS patients—
before one, two, then three or more combination therapies came into play.

DOCSPEAK 201: ADVANCES

"The truth is…it's incremental advancement," Venook went on to tell me
during our interview. Then he mentioned two newish chemo drugs,
irinotecan (Camptosar), and oxaliplatin, that survivors should get to
know, just in case. They're part of the new palette, but not as newswor-
thy (recently) as Avastin and Erbitux. For a moment I was surprised at his
blunt candor. Then I remembered: He always was the toughest-talking
doctor on my team (and my team included Dr. Peter Carroll, urologic surgeon at UCSF, who in 2000 was chosen to treat and operate on Robert
Mueller, our nation's FBI chief). Then again, as I write this while in complete remission, I have no quibble with his…results.

The best ways to turn hope into long-term survival, Venook and his colleagues believe, will become evident when more genetic codes are
cracked; and when dozens more clinical trials (such as Holper's) are com-
pleted. "Question is, Can you find patients…who are truly curable?"
Venook asks. "We have known for some years, for example, that the liver
is the most common site of recurrence for colorectal cancers. And back in
the '70s and '80s, this recurrence used to be deemed just a horrible thing.
Now our group (and I'm including researchers at Memorial Sloan-
Kettering in New York and M.D. Anderson [in Houston]) has found that
we can actually cure those who've had METS to the liver. They've been
cured, after five years. It's no bargain, to be sure, this spread of the cancer. But while it's not good, there is a subset of patients, where it may be
the only place that it has spread, that now are cured."

In fact, for some survivors who have endured one, two or more courses of
chemo, and who still have new or recurrent lesions on their liver, a new
laser-surgery procedure called Radio Frequency Ablation (RFA) may help

achieve remission. While gaining in popularity at leading colon cancer research centers, RFA doesn't yet achieve what Venook and his colleagues ultimately are aiming for: known, knockout punches. But it is helping them get closer—and buying all-important time, which now means years, instead of months, of extended life.

THE PATIENT'S EDGE (Part IV)

In Fred Holper's case, he hadn't had RFA treatments by the time we first spoke; he was focused on other events: My fiancée said, when I came home from surgery and the hospital, 'I want you to promise me, if the CAT scan is fine, and numbers aren't screwed... I want to get married.' I said, 'You thought I was nuts? Now which part of this don't you understand? I'm gonna die.' Then I [calmed down and] said, 'If the CAT scan is fine, AND everything is okay...we can do it. So I come home; all still seemed fine. So she said, 'I want to get married.' We got married October 25th. I got my next chemo 'holiday' for 4 weeks. We went to Europe; got married over there. Then I went right back on this stuff.'"

Still, Holper knew: His may not, ultimately, be a happily-ever-after story. But it was a happily-hitched-then tale, a happily-longer-than-anybody-dared-to-hope tale. It is, to many in the colorectal cancer community, awe-inspiring stuff.

"After my second cycle of Avastin, after 14 weeks from surgery, we were down [the tumors were down] 70 percent in size, by my oncologist's calipers. I thought they might disappear altogether. Didn't happen. At end of first year of treatments, January of '02—after one year—I decided to go with my medical friends on a mercenary visit to Guatemala, to bring down first aid and general care. People said, 'You're nuts. You have terminal cancer and you're going to a third world country.' I said: '*You* don't understand. It was my family; my in-laws, who were the ones saying I was nuts.

"The way I saw it, I wasn't supposed to be here after a year. So I want to live life on my terms. 'But what if something happens to you down there?,' they said. I said I had practically my whole surgical team down there with me.... So I was adamant about that.

"The two reasons I [have survived so long]," Holper told me, "talking to you [today], in no particular order, are: my faith—that there is a greater Authority, a greater good; and, obviously, the Avastin. And I wouldn't put my faith in God before the Avastin. I'm not a Bible thumper. I'm a reasonably mainstream Christian. For some reason, He wanted me to stay alive; He gave me the ability to get into this study, on this drug, and survive."

NEWSFLASH!

"THE NEXT NEW THING...
IN COLORECTAL SCREENING"

Seeing is relieving. Especially when the viewing involves the large intestine, is less painful than prior methods, quicker, and just as accurate.

For countless patients at risk for colon cancer or recurrence, the traditional scope colonoscopy, which remains quite effective as the current "gold standard" in screening in North America, now faces new, high-tech-video competition—called "virtual colonoscopy."

In fact, an article in the *New England Journal of Medicine* in late 2003, brought a startling finding: After studying more than 1,200 low-risk subjects for colon cancer, researchers from the University of Wisconsin medical school found the methods "equally" accurate in locating polyps during a standard screening. One of two malignant polyps, however, that were discovered during the study, was missed by the traditional endoscopic (scope) colonoscopy. That's not to say (not yet, anyway) that the new, CAT-scan tests, which use forced air and computers to make pictures of exactly what's inside the colon, are more effective, overall, than colonoscopy.

What is important, however, is that in certain cases, virtual colonoscopy offers proven advantages in screening. Because the test takes half the time of a colonoscopy, more patients may opt to use the test. Which may mean more early detection. On the other hand, doctors tend to use less (or no) sedation during these exams, so patients may actually feel more pain during a "virtual" look, than a twisting, flexible scope-with-mini-camera attached at the front end. And both exams require fasting, bowel cleansing, and laxatives the day before the exam, to allow docs to see literally everything in your large intestine.

There are, to be sure, other ways to look. Today, the two even-less-invasive tests for colon cancer—stool-blood swab home tests, and genetic testing of stool samples collected at home by patients and sent to labs—are gaining favor. So too, is new testing for mutations (alterations) in a colon cancer-related gene called KRAS—an advance highlighted by experts at the 2008 ASCO annual meeting of clinical oncologists. This gene test helps determine if the drugs Erbitux or Vectibix can be effective in later-stage treatment. And all these tests will likely continue to increase their "reach" over the next 5 to10 years. For it may take that long to verify the reliability, and safety, of the virtual and genetic exams, the Next New Thing in colorectal screening.

Dental EFX: One More Reason Chemo Bites

When you're fighting a life-threatening cancer, let's be honest, you don't always find time to floss. I found that out the hard way, more than 2 years after my colon cancer surgery, when I learned I was facing a root canal, at age 46, the first of my rather mainstream dental career. Though they were both polite and professional, the staff at North Boulder Dental Center in Colorado basically told me I had no choice. 'Twasn't a normal cavity in one of my bottom-right-quadrant molars. It was a nasty one that was reaching and twiddling the nerve. I wasn't happy, to be sure, but I was intrigued when the hygienist told me that while chemotherapy may save your life, it dries up your mouth terribly. And a dry tongue, cheek and gums, it turns out, over time, leads to cavities way more often than comparably moist oral tissues found in healthy people. Wish I would've known that three years ago....

MARTHA STEWART'S ANTI-CANCER RECIPE

Don't get me wrong.... I'm not one of those protestors who stood outside of Manhattan's Federal Courthouse on Centre Street with a sign that read "FREE MARTHA" during the end stages of Martha Stewart's ImClone stock trial in mid-2004. Nor do I think she should have been set free (after allegedly lying to federal prosecutors during an investigation of illicit stock trading) due to her status and accomplishments. But as a colon cancer patient-turned-survivor it seems I can't *not* make at least two points:

1) Whatever the reason[s] Stewart sold her 3,928 shares of ImClone in December 2001, the fact remains: It was Stewart and people like her, along with, yes, major institutional investors, who plunked down serious cash for stock in a pharmaceutical company early on that had no guarantee of success in beating advanced colon cancer tumors. The company took on major financial risks in order to research new medicines and eventually prolong the lives of colorectal cancer patients. In this case, investors like Martha Stewart, let's face it: whether you like her or avoid her, weren't

throwing money at a "hot" new tech stock; or jamming to invest in the initial public offering of (extremely high-carb) Krispy Kreme doughnuts.

2) Whatever the reason[s] Stewart allegedly lied about her financial dealings, the fact remains: I am glad, extremely glad, Erbitux is an option for me to try, should my adenocarcinoma some day return....

Modern Treatments-At-a-Glance

The news is striking: Of the chemotherapy and biological-based drugs listed below, six have been FDA-approved for use since 2002 in the U.S. or by the European Medicines Agency (EMA). Prior to these approvals, most oncologists had just one or two, maybe three, combinations of chemo to offer patients with which they felt familiar. Times have changed. In a hurry. In a way, what's happening in colorectal cancer treatments today echoes what's happened with treatments for HIV/AIDS and breast cancer over the past 20 years. Doctors and researchers are now trying new combinations of colon cancer drugs—including oral chemo meds (from the likes of Sanofi, Merck)—to try to outsmart the disease, finally.

And while most patients and survivors instantly think of "drugs" when they talk of treatment, they have in recent years begun to broaden their thinking, experts say. Here's why: Not only has a new host of colorectal cancer medicines come to market, but radiation treatment has improved for rectal cancer patients; and surgery, too (including RFA and even newer, Evident® microwave ablation for liver tumors) has become more far successful since 2000. The news doesn't stop there: Integrative medicine (combining modern methods with herbal or nutritional therapies) has moved into more mainstream cancer treatment and made itself a key adjunct, whereas it used to be mostly considered as an afterthought.

"The liver is the most common site of recurrence," says Alan Venook, M.D., of University of California-San Francisco's (UCSF) cancer center. Now, in part because of advances in genetic-based medicines, he says, "we can point to those who are cured after five years."   [SEE NEXT PAGE FOR TREATMENTS]

COMMON TREATMENTS IN THE U.S.

Treatment (trade name)	Firm	How it Works	Type of Drug	Comments
fluorouracil; also called 5-FU under multiple trade names	Mayne Pharma; multiple makers	Kills cancer cells systemically by interfering with their reproduction. Often paired with luecovorin, a vitaminlike enhancing agent.	Chemo	Used in chemo "cocktails" like FOLFOX, FOLFIRI; in stronger, multicombinations than were available soon after 2000.
capecitabine (Xeloda®)	Hoffman-LaRoche/ Roche	An "anti-metabolite," this is taken orally and converts to 5-FU in the body; No IVneeded, which points to lifestyle advantages, fewer trips to infusion centers.	Oral oncology pill	Prescribed for metastatic colorectal and breast cancers. May cause "hand and foot" syndrome (rash) side-EFX; anemia
irinotecan (Camptosar®)	Pfizer Oncology; patent expired in 2008, leading to generic forms	Blocks enzymes from helping cells to divide. Is administered by IV; also paired with 5-FU and leucovorin in combo called FOLFIRI.	Chemo	Has been shown to delay tumor growth markedly; FDA approved 1998. Used against recurrent or spread metastatic colorectal cancer in combination with other agents. Is the "IRI" in FOLFIRI.
oxaliplatin (Eloxatin®)	Sanofi-Aventis	Known as the sticky chemo, this platimum-based med works against the very DNA of cancer cells, causing cell destruction.	Chemo	FDA approved with expanded access (including FOLFOX4), '02; also used in chemo 'cocktails,' Stage III
cetuximab (Erbitux®)	ImClone/ Lilly in U.S.; Merck in Europe/Asia	Monoclonal antibody, meaning it "hunts" tumor cells and delivers fatal blows to the cancer growth factors, without harming normal, surrounding cells.	Biologic	FDA-OK'd Feb 2004, for Stage IV colon cancers. May be less-debilitating than other approved cocan meds, yet requires certain KRAS-gene typing for efficacy.
bevacizumab (Avastin®)	Genentech	As a so-called targeted drug ("angiogenesis inhibitor,"), it starves tumors by robbing them of blood vessel agents needed to grow.	Biologic, with fewer side-EFX than many chemo drugs	FDA-approved, Feb. 2004 for Stage IV colon cancers; used with 'FOLFOX' combo treatments.

TREATMENTS TO WATCH: PROMISING PROSPECTS

The following new therapies for various stages of colorectal cancer are in new phases of treatment (or in clinical trials) throughout North America or Europe. Some may make it to the wider marketplace fairly soon.

Treatment (trade or temporary name)	Maker	How it Works	Comments
panitumumab (Vectibix®)	Amgen	Monoclonal antibody; targets EGFR, or epidermal growth factor receptors in tumors, halting or slowing spread.	FDA-approved in 2006 for secondline treatment of advanced CoCan; certain gene factors (KRAS gene) greatly affect its efficacy.
pemetrexed (Altima®)	Eli Lilly	A cytotoxic agent that breaks the chain of folat-edependent cell metabo-lism. Delays certain cancer cells from replication	FDA-OK'd for some lung cancers; but has shown strong activity against advanced colorectal cancers in combo with Eloxatin* therapy.
PTK787 (Vatalanib®)	Novartis/ Schering	Another angiogenesis inhibitor, may have poten-tial to become an Avastin*-like treatment, in cutting tumors' blood supply.	Used as secondline drug in advanced cases. Recent studies tested it as add-on to oxaliplatin/5-FU /leucovorin as well.
tegafur-uracil (UFT®)	Merck KGaA	Oral chemo, an antimetabo-lite. Tegafur is a 5-FU "pro-drug" that converts to 5-FU in the body; uracil slows its breakdown to extend drug's effects.	Beyond colon and rectal tumors, in new tests against breast, pancreatic and other cancers. Cost savings vs. IVdrugs may spur wide acceptance in U.S. and Europe.
CyberKnife®	Accuray	Uses focused radiation delivered via photon beams and a robotic arm. Often used in colon cancer tumors that have spread to brain.	Actually uses no "knife" or scalpel; can help progression free survival when surgery isn't advised. Is related to GammaKnife, which came before.
SIR-Spheres®	Sirtex	Mini-micro beads (polymer-coated) of radiation sent via portal vein directly into liver, without coursing through rest of body.	Used experimentally when previous rounds of chemo/bio haven't succeed-ed; also when liver metastases are few.
RadioFrequency Ablation (RFA)	Varian; RITA Medical Systems	Destroys colon cancer tumor tissue that's spread to liver or lung by "super-heating" soft tissue around RFA elec-trode. (Most stage IV CoCan cases advance to liver.)	Can be administered via needle guide to tumor through the skin; or in open surgery, if docs see better odds of killing tumor directly using that access point. RFA can be repeated; surgery option may still follow.

CHAPTER 5

Holistic Health Help: Complementary & Alternative Therapies

So far, so good. Pop pill. Swallow. Swish of water... slightly chalky aftertaste. Nearly four years since my Stage III diagnosis and now? NED, as the experts say...No Evidence of Disease. So what's with the pill?

The last time I spent money to fight colon cancer—using cash instead of a Blue Shield health insurance card or personal check for a doctor co-pay—I dropped $12.99 at Walgreens for a bottle of 500 generic aspirin tabs. Nothing fancy, not too high tech. Nothing too dicey in terms of side effects (due to my low-strength, 81 milligram tablets, one every other day, rather than the 500 mg "extra-strength" version). In sum, nothing too complex by way of drug delivery or pharmacology.

" The most important element to survival is adaptability, the ability to change your goals and needs. The second-most important element to survival is a positive outlook.... "

– Mark Burnett, television producer, *Survivor*, and combat war veteran, Falkland Islands conflict, as told to *Esquire*.

And yet, I may be doing myself some real good, even though I am assuming a small risk (as all drugs have side effects) here. Yes, there has been scientific proof that aspirin can help prevent heart disease, heart attack and stroke, in part by helping to keep the bloodstream running smoothly. There's even been evidence that aspirin—a 100+ year-old drug—can help save lives as emergency medicine, when taken immediately by those who have suffered a heart attack in public, and who are awaiting paramedics. (Always a good idea to carry a travel pack in your purse or briefcase.) Still, blood that's too thin may at times be unhealthful; and we're still waiting for iron-clad proof that low-grade, regular dose aspirin will prevent colorectal cancer...or its recurrence.

TAKE TWO ASPIRIN...AND CALL ME IN FIVE YEARS

We are, however, getting closer. Much closer. Back in 1991, a key American Cancer Society study followed more than 650,000 men and women (nearly 10 football stadiums' capacity) who ingested as few as 16 aspirin tablets a month, roughly every other day, like me. They found, in short, that this group had a 40 percent reduced colon cancer mortality rate compared to what might have been expected, without aspirin. Not 4, nor 14 percent...but 40 percent! The researchers were pleased, maybe even stunned, but cautioned that it was "too soon" to advise all those concerned about colon cancer to begin taking low-dose aspirin regularly. Later, a different reputable study looked at aspirin use among those who are prone to develop polyps of the colon (which can progress to cancer), and showed significant protective effects. And, much more recently, (in 2004), research from Columbia University in New York helped tip my personal scale of secondary prevention.

These newer findings, published that summer in the *Journal of the American Medical Association*, didn't exactly apply to me: They came from a study of more than 2,800 women, half of whom had breast cancer;

half of whom were healthy. I fully realize that, molecularly-speaking, breast cancer and colon cancer cells are wholly different animals. And many of us know that chemotherapy for one cancer usually doesn't simply transfer to another. But the *JAMA* report was a well-designed trial that showed those who took aspirin daily were 28 percent less likely to develop breast cancer than those who didn't take aspirin. Also, those who took aspirin only once (!) a week were 20 percent less likely to eventually have breast cancer, compared to those who took no aspirin. These are big numbers; something clearly is going on here.

Due to these two human, and "more than a hundred animal studies" since the 1980s, according to Mark Bennett Pochapin, M.D., of New York-Presbyterian Hospital-Weill Cornell Medical School, I decided to become an aspirin guinea pig, of sorts. (But first, I ran it by my oncologist.) My doc didn't encourage me to take this "complementary" medicine; but he didn't discourage me, either, as we await... (the researchers' fave refrain) "more specific studies." When we realized I don't have stomach ulcers nor tend to suffer other gastro bleeding, which aspirin can cause, he gave me a knowing nod, stopping a bit short of an endorsement.

Still, there are times in every cancer patient's, or survivor's, life when he or she decides to decide *now*, instead of waiting for more studies. This one seemed safe enough, prudent enough, for me. Especially as it may help prevent heart disease as well. As I write this, I'm 46, not 36. Can't help but think, more often than I used to, about how my heart, and not just my intestines, will hold up over time.

TRACKING NEW DRUG TRIALS

When making decisions about what's new that may also be right for you, it helps to know a bit about those who've been there before. Here are four reputable sources for reports about clinical trials of new drugs, new agents or new combinations of the same:

- The Colon Cancer Alliance (877-422-2030)
  www.ccalliance.org/patients_trials_finding.html

- Oncolink @ University of Pennsylvania Medical Center
  www.oncolink.org/treatment (800-789-PENN) (7366)

- Coalition of National Cancer Cooperative Groups, Inc. (877.520.4457)
  www.CancerTrialsHelp.org

- (NCCAM) The National Center for Complementary and Alternative
  Medicine, National Institutes of Health (888.644.6226)
  www.nccam.nih.gov

CLOVE AT FIRST SIGHT: GOING GARLIC

Not long ago, I needed a new prescription of sorts. Feeling more New Age-healthful than usual, I hopped on my bike (to help preserve the atmosphere's ozone layer) and pedaled over to the Boulder, Colorado headquarters of the Herb Research Foundation (HRF), passing a few notable buildings along the way…. In less than a half-mile, I rolled by the Sensenig Chiropractic Center; the adobe-style, kibbutz-like, Nomad Co-housing Community; a firm called EcoFutures; and the well-manicured home of a neighbor who wrote a book called *Energy Revolution.* I went to the HRF to get some advice about garlic; to find out how such an old gritty bulb has slowly, surely, come to be seen in a new light. (I had ordered the info online, but I was in search of hard copies.)

What I found made me rethink my long-term, anti-tumor arsenal. I'd long known of the pro-cardiac and antimicrobial properties of garlic, and how World War I soldiers used it in Europe on their wounds…but it was news to me that garlic is also considered a cholesterol reducer, and that, in Europe, people already use it, with doctors' approval, to prevent cancer. Including colon cancer. As the HRF folks put it: "Perhaps the world's best example of a medicinal food, garlic is one of the most intensively studied herbs in natural medicine today."

Sparing you (most of) the details, I'll share here the best bits of what my $7.00 purchase of HRF-reviewed research materials contained about garlic:

- lowers the risk of colon and stomach cancer

- arrests the activity of "cancer-causing substances"

- may inhibit tumor formation and protect against damage from chemotherapy and radiation

- a study of 41,000 Iowa women found that those who ate garlic at least once each week reduced the risk of colon cancer by 35 percent. (results published in *American Journal of Epidemiology* in 1994)

- clinical studies showed garlic tablets (containing high-quality garlic powder) were effective at a dose of 600 to 900 mg per day

This, mostly, is why a bottle of Garlicin (a leading brand made by Nature's Way) garlic powder tablets now stands at attention in my kitchen cabinet, betwixt my bottles of Solgar Advanced Antioxidant Formula supplements and my Allergy Research make of CoQ10 enzyme pills.

If you're too far to bike, you might try the HRF at:
www.herbs.org/herbinfopack.html

STATINS STATS: NOT JUST FOR CHOLESTEROL...

At first I was skeptical: After all, the news was from New Orleans, where shady things have been known to happen, day or night.... This time, though, it was a potentially major finding for colon cancer survivors, promoted at an annual cancer research conference in mid-2004. As it turns out, scientists studied statins—the cholesterol-lowering "wonder" drugs—in nearly 4,000 people and found a significant, protective benefit against colorectal cancer and maybe other cancers as well....

In a brief summary: The study of statins such as Lipitor, Zocar and Prevachol, in those who are prone to colon cancer, showed the drugs might reduce a subject's colon cancer risk by as much as half—a stunning 50 percent drop.

Stephen Gruber, M.D., of the University of Michigan's Cancer Center, called the data "very exciting," even though it was not-yet-final. Fact was, according to a reporter who attended the American Society of Clinical Oncologists meeting, it was the largest study ever of its kind. That's enough information, I'd say, to at least remember prescription "statins" as a possible chemo-preventive in one's long-term market basket of "maybes."

100 WORDS ABOUT YOGA

The recent newspaper story said: "Many Americans who have cancer have rushed through their daily grind..." until cancer wreaked havoc in their lives. The story also said, "A growing number of hospitals are discovering a tranquil, 5,000 year-old therapy from India that may help them—yoga."

"It's the oldest strategy for stress management," according to Debra Mulnick, a nurse who offers classes at St. Luke's Regional Medical Center in Boise. Some sages, even older than yoga itself, might argue her point and counter: "No, death is the oldest strategy for stress management."

Not that there's anything right with that.

MEDICAL MARIJUANA, LEGALIZED (Part I)

In 1996, California voters passed Proposition 215 allowing for the sale and medical use of marijuana for patients with AIDS, cancer, and other serious and painful diseases. Nine other states later followed suit.

MEDICAL MARIJUANA LEGALIZED (Part II)

An excerpt from my wife, Paula's, journal, sharing a caregiver's view of my (licensed) marijuana use, over seven months' time, in '01:

When I went to buy pot for Curt [in San Francisco], it reminded me of a chemo center. I remember watching a report on the news [on the medical marijuana 'store'] but the cameras didn't go inside. It seemed like a bar from the outside; I imagined it would feel like a bar, after I saw the report....

Then I went inside: It was set up kind of like a shop. There were tables, people who worked there were professional sounding; straight. People were sitting down along one wall in there and these were all terribly sick, bald (I remember a bald woman in there) patients. All of a sudden it didn't feel like—there was no party going on—it felt more like a pharmacy. I mean, the guy who worked behind the counter started asking me about Curt's symptoms: Did he need it more for nausea, or pain? Pain where? There were different kinds, different grades.

There was a limit to how much you could buy; they checked your IDs carefully. I believe there was a private room upstairs, with a clergyman, for counseling. You couldn't bring a friend inside; you had to be a card-carrying member. Everyone in there was a patient or a caregiver. I can't imagine...it's got to be

better than taking morphine, which the doctors said, was the next step for Curt
if he couldn't get his pain under control. We were told that was the next step.

MEDICAL MARIJUANA LEGALIZED (Part III)

In 2004, the U.S. Supreme Court agreed to hear a case, filed by Ms. Angel
Raich, 38, of Oakland, against the federal government's alleged mishan-
dling of California's Proposition 215. The case stems from a controversial Drug Enforcement Agency raid, which was intent on confiscating six
marijuana plants from a (licensed) patient's private land in rural
California. Raich, according to her doctor, suffers from an inoperable
brain tumor.

ACUPUNCTURE EFX

In Hollywood, they like to use the shorthand "EFX" for the word
"effects," as in special, or visual EFX. Old film tricks have become updated into hip, techno-cinematic tools. These days in Cancerland, acupuncture is getting a new look, one with more seasoned, and international,
respect. Old healing tricks from China that call for "needling" the body in
pain points and target tissues have been updated into "hot" techno-med-
ical tools.

But unlike flashy whiz-bang in the movies, the acupuncture EFX upon
the body have both temporary and lasting value. Acupuncture, as practiced in modern America, goes well beyond relieving back and neck pain.
In fact, the landmark year was 1997, when a National Institutes of Health
panel proclaimed there was solid evidence of benefit from acupuncture
for relief of nausea and vomiting due to surgery, chemotherapy and child-
birth. The experts also pointed to acupuncture's potential to bring
migraine relief, possibly counter addiction, and reduce low-back pain,
though data was less sufficient in these areas.

Bottom line was—and is—acupuncture has the potential to help cancer patients or survivors on two levels:

1) Pain relief: which can help patients reduce long-term load of opiates or other pain relievers.

2) Relaxation: patients often heal more quickly and completely when fully relaxed, a state which often occurs after a 30-minute needle treatment session.

We're not talking cancer cure, here, but an additional treatment that apparently works on multiple levels. When I talked with Barrie Cassileth, Ph.D., the head of the integrative medical therapy at Memorial Sloan-Kettering Cancer Center in New York City, about what complementary healing modalities patients use frequently at MSK, she mentioned acupuncture, yoga, massage and guided imagery (visualization), as four top complementary therapies. What I found most memorable about Cassileth's take on acupuncture was that scientists for years have thought the reported benefits of acupuncture were "imagined." That's no longer the case.

"We used to think the gains [of acupuncture] were due to a placebo effect," Cassileth says, "but that can't be said to be true for children and animal studies, and they have both shown positive effects." (When it comes to lab studies, animals simply have no way to "fake" feeling better.) She cites new scans, known as functional MRI, which can track brain changes caused by any number of behaviors...including getting medically stuck by needles to dampen pain and promote healing.

MY EXPERIMENTAL MOMENTS

In my case, I'd met with an acupuncturist, but didn't sign up before I found a certain Rosemary. Or , should I say, Rosemary found me?....

All I wanted was a break from the pain. In the long run, of course, I wanted more: I wanted the cancer causing my pain to die. Meantime, six weeks after a diagnosis of malignant disease that was ceaselessly attacking my rectum and ceaselessly sending shock waves up my spinal cord, I was flat on my back on a couch four-to-six hours a day. While waiting hours each day for various opiods to kick in and blunt the hurt, I remember moaning in agony, crying because I'd run out of ways to suck-it-up. I recall wondering how a silent-for-so-long disease could prove so wicked-nasty-powerful. Then one afternoon, I heard the doorbell ring downstairs.

Up to that point, I felt I'd done everything right in my course of treatment. "Yes," I'd said, to postponing my surgery for three months shortly after diagnosis, so my docs and I could "front-load" my tumor with more chemo and radiation, two months before the planned operation. This approach was still considered experimental at the time by many, because in the Old Days (up till the early-to-mid 1990s), the standard operating procedure, literally, was to go in and get-the-cancer-the-heck-outa-there: What were we, what was I, waiting for?

Actually, by treating me with six weeks of chemotherapy plus radiation pre-operatively, to shrink the tumor and operating "field," my doctors at University of California-San Francisco (UCSF) believed I would have a better surgical outcome, and a better chance of remission and full cure. My tumor was in a tricky spot, they said, lodged in my rectum down deep in the pelvis, dangerously close to the prostate gland. To operate immediately after diagnosis might, at first thought, have made me feel like a more aggressive, in-control patient. So I'd have scored psyche points. (And in fact, one doctor in the Midwest went ahead and scheduled my surgery for three weeks after I got my diagnosis, without offering me a chance at pre-op chemo-radiation.) Looking back, I didn't vote that way. And, as I said, the doorbell rang....

MY LEFT FOOT: AN ACUPRESSURE "MIRACLE"

I didn't want to visit with our friend Rosemary, frankly. As soothing as her voice has always been to Paula, I was a sad sack of guy, not feeling conversational or in the least bit social. But she walked in, and approached my diseased body carefully. She sat down beside it on the couch, and lightly wrapped her fingers around my toes and the ball of my foot. She started pushing and probing the underside of my foot; then harder, doing things with small bones I didn't know existed inside my sole.... Suddenly she wasn't merely Paula's pal. She was Rosemary Shoong, energy healer whom I remembered had studied alternative therapies in both Europe and the U.S.

Within 10-to-15 minutes, pain began to *whoosh* through my legs...down through pipes, it felt like, down my legs and out my ankles and the heels of my feet...whooshing fast and shooting out in an instant, forgetting that I had toes.

To this day, Rosemary Shoong's impromptu, ultra-reflexology of sorts remains a mystery to me. It wasn't just the pain relief that stayed with me, for I'd experienced Big Gun killers like Vicodin, pot and other opiods.... It was the power of what she did with touch, with pressure, with healing techniques that had been passed to her and practiced, for centuries, not mere decades.

Rosemary didn't simply open my eyes to alternative medical cancer treatment. She opened my world, figuratively and literally. It was energy healing, therapeutic touch, at full, measured, throttle. Now I sit comfortably, three-plus years later, silently wishing, praying (sometimes at night, while all alone) that I never have to feel that bad to feel so good, again.

CAM: A SURVIVORS' SHORT COURSE

In plotting a course through or beyond chemotherapy and recovery, you may want to tailor your long-term strategies to include one or a few of the above complementary or alternative medical (CAM) therapies. If so, there are more than a few federal medical libraries and experts worth consulting for advice…and from which these following five points emerge. I consider them a conservative view of liberal-minded medical regimens:

- Many patients and consumers believe that "natural" means safe. Not necessarily so. Wild mushrooms, for instance, can be safe to eat, while other wild mushrooms are deadly. Caveat: choose and chew carefully.

- Ask the maker or marketer of a new(-ish) CAM nutrient, drug or supplement, for any science-minded articles or the results of key studies. They should be willing to share e-links or hard copies quickly.

- Contact a nearby medical school or hospital to ask if they post lists of area CAM practitioners. If not, ask if they could recommend a patient advocate who is familiar with CAM, or a nurse or physician assistant who has oncology/complementary medicine experience.

- Antioxidant vitamins and nutrients, while helpful, affect countless cells in the body…and may affect how well (or poorly) chemotherapy does its job. Chemo tries to kill millions of cells; antioxidants sometimes prevent cells from dying. A tricky mix to manage at times.

- Be suspicious of claims that purportedly cure a wide range of unrelated disorders (i.e., cancer, diabetes, and AIDS). No product can treat every disease and condition.

Almost goes without saying, but cancer patients and survivors need to discuss information about CAM with their health care provider(s) before making any decisions about new treatments.

For more information:

NCCAM Clearinghouse
National Institutes of Health
P.O. Box 7923
Gaithersburg, MD 20898-7923
888.644.6226
301.519.3153
866.464.3615 TTY (for hard-of-hearing)
866.464.3616 Fax
www.nccam.nih.gov
www.nlm.nih.gov/nccam/camonpubmed.html (for journal links)

Green Tea...Stirs up Trouble?

After years of pro-health messages about green tea, it might be time to
"bag it," and hold off—at least during certain chemotherapy rounds,
experts recently found. In a startling 2008 study conducted at the Keck
School of Medicine at USC near Los Angeles, researchers discovered that
EGCG, a component of green tea extract, actually interfered with the anti-
cancer effects of the cancer drug, Velcade, in experimental mice with
tumors. "Our finding that... EGCG blocked the therapeutic action of
Velcade was completely unexpected," said Axel H. Schonthal, Ph.D.,
study author and associate professor in microbiology and immunology at
USC. Although the cancer drug in question here was FDA-approved for
multiple myeloma (a blood cancer), and not colorectal cancer, the study's
impact could be far-reaching. In fact, I first learned of it on a colon cancer (www.fightcolorectalcancer.org) Website. Still, one study (of mice)
doesn't mean green tea doesn't provide key health benefits throughout life
for humans: It simply means cancer patients, for now, should be aware of
tea-and-complementary medicine alerts, both pro and con, when asking
their docs about "what else" to take to bolster their long-term arsenal.

The Anti-Cancer Cheeseburger?

You want sweet-potato fries with that? Don't look now, but our government is growing cattle that have been bred—and fed—to some day be able to produce, for us, anti-cancer cheeseburgers.

The thinking goes like this: Selenium, a nutrient and naturally abundant mineral, happens to have healthful, antioxidant properties. (Which means, like vitamins A, C, E and CoQ10, it helps neutralize "free-radical" molecules in our blood that carry extra oxygen electrons and have the potential to trigger aging and diseases, including cancer.) So if we know high-fat, frequent cheeseburger diets contribute to heart disease and sometimes colon cancer, what if we fortify the cow? How about we let cattle graze on selenium-rich land, for months or years, in order to produce meat that has anti-cancer agents, in a sense, already "built-in?" The thinking also goes: To many people, this would be more "natural" than injecting vitamins or nutrients directly into cattle, or simply lacing the feed with selenium supplements.

"These foods will be fed to laboratory animals to determine the protective effects of selenium against cancer," say scientists with the U.S. Department of Agriculture research service, who planned to analyze the pilot project in late 2004. "Foods will also be fed to humans living in a low-selenium area...."

Yeah, I'll take fries with that. And a follow-up CT scan in five years.

CHAPTER 6

How to Eat to Live Longer

On one hand, Dr. Nixon's words at right make terrific sense. You can't wholly blame your cancer on your diet; nor are 10 servings of veggies a day enough to ensure a cancer-free future. A sensible, hopeful middle ground. Plus, you want to be*lieve* someone like Dr. Nixon, who has served as both director of cancer prevention at the Medical University of South Carolina and as a vice-president of detection and treatment at the American Cancer Society. On the other hand, as a patient, survivor or family member who's dealt with the disease, you have to ask: If food isn't *that* important in the battle against cancer recurrence, why did Doc Nixon fill 425 pages of a book with advice about eating to help control or conquer the disease?

At one point he tells patients, "Try to become at least a part-time vegetarian, and gradually

" Nutrition…is not the sole cause of any cancer, nor is nutrition alone an effective treatment. [But] good nutrition with other factors can contribute to cancer-risk reduction and the chances of cancer remission. "

– Daniel W. Nixon, M.D.,
oncologist and author,
The Cancer Recovery Eating Plan

increase the number of meat-free meals you have each week." At another he suggests to those at risk for colorectal cancer: "It is also a good idea to increase your consumption of the garlic-family vegetables and foods rich in beta-carotene [including broccoli, cantaloupe, butternut squash, kale, sweet potatoes, spinach]. There's got to be something compelling and powerful about the food/cancer connection; something perhaps stronger than Nixon's strict scientific background has allowed him to publicly support.

I found it, or part of it, in his last chapter, known as "The Program," which can be summed up in five steps:

1) Reduce dietary fat
2) Increase consumption of dietary fiber
3) Emphasize foods that contain "chemopreventive agents" [Nixon's term] that have been shown to be effective against certain cancers (at least in animal studies)
4) Eat a variety of nutritious foods daily
5) Make moderate, regular exercise a priority; as it has many health benefits and may help reduce cancer risk.

The news Nixon brings isn't that he, like other experts, stresses fiber and less fat, but that he believes wholeheartedly many foods, eaten often and wisely, can deliver chemopreventive benefits. In my mind, that makes food—combined with regular exercise—a form of medicine. Of course, not all medicines work for all patients. Yet most of them do, which is why I've started eating (and drinking) differently since my diagnosis and recovery. As I wrote in my journal months after my surgery…

PULP FRICTION

Whirrrr-chop-chop-vrruuuuuuuhhhh!!! Got a juicer the other week, a bona fide institutional kind that weighs a ton, cost nearly $300, and grinds the goodness out of pretty much anything that grows on trees or out of the ground. *Vruhhhh-chop.* There's no scientific proof of freshly extracted juice adding 6.2 years to my life or anything; just advice from a good friend from Tulsa and a reasoned attempt to keep things that shouldn't be growing inside me from growing inside me.

CHART TOPPER

On a (slightly) more scientific note, two physicians from the famed Memorial Sloan-Kettering Cancer Center in New York published a chart in their book, *Cancer Free: The Comprehensive Prevention Program*, that, once you've seen it, is not easy to forget (an abridged version follows). It strikes a powerful image of what some doctors think is a critical link— between diet and cancers. But that doesn't mean they know how exactly to prevent the disease through better eating. We're all still learning:

A POST-MORTEM ON HOW CANCER GROWS *

Cause	% of Cancer Deaths
Diet	35%
Tobacco use	30%
Reproductive + Sexual Behavior	7%
Occupational Hazards	4%
Excessive Alcohol	3%
Excessive Sun Exposure	3%
Environmental Pollution	2%

Source: "Cancer Free" by Sidney J. Winawer, M.D. and Moshe Shike, M.D. (2000, Simon & Schuster)

* Note: As chart is abridged for clarity, rows above do not add to 100 percent. Remaining 16 percent is spread among numerous factors.

GOT YOGURT?

So now we know, or have been reminded, that food has a cameo-if-not-featured role in preventing recurrence. So now we ask: How far should we go toward using it in our defense? The answer is decidedly personal. But if each patient thinks of diet as part of the arsenal, and acts positively, he or she should benefit to some degree.

An example: Not long ago, *The American Journal of Clinical Nutrition* ran an important article entitled, "Yogurt and Gut Function." To be honest, I don't read this journal often (it mostly goes to dietitians), but something was nagging at me that sent me there: A former doctor of mine, a world-renowned New York oncologist, had written and spoken about the need for extra calcium in the fight to prevent colorectal cancer. So you'd think: Simple, drink more milk. Yet I also remembered that in 2000 in England, where I lived at the time, professor Jane Plant had published a controversial book, *Your Life is in Your Hands*, which drew disturbing links between dairy products and breast cancer.

Plant, a breast cancer survivor, went so far as to report, "Then I eliminated dairy products. Within days, the lump started to shrink.... I now believe that the link between dairy produce and breast cancer (and probably prostate cancer) is similar to that between smoking and lung cancer." In the U.S., where the multi-million-dollar "Got Milk?" ad campaign had run for months in major media outlets, Plant's book, perhaps not surprisingly, didn't get nearly as much publicity as in the U.K. (save for an article about it in the likes of American *Elle*, the fashion magazine). I was left to wonder: If both experts are correct, could milk products help control colon cancer, but also help cause breast cancer? Maybe it's the kind of milk product that's key....

The authors of the yogurt article in *The American Journal* didn't try to boldly say that eating a tub of Dannon a day will keep colon cancer at bay. Instead they summarized dozens of reputable studies on yogurt and human physiology and concluded there were numerous links between eating certain kinds of yogurt and lower incidence of colon cancer. In short, we've long known that antibiotics can kill bacteria. What we're now learning is that "probiotics," like the good bacteria found in certain yogurts, can help keep selected cells from turning harmful inside our intestines. To wit: "...the feeding of yogurt or *Lactobacillus* reduced fecal enzymes, which convert procarcinogens to carcinogens...." One translation of this might be that in *some* bodies, yogurt actually slows the process of pre-cancerous activity. It delays the process by which potentially lethal cells would otherwise become lethal.

Bottom line: Double chocolate frozen yogurt (with sprinkles) at the food court probably won't do the trick. High-quality yogurts, however, that boast lactobacillus bacteria on the label, may be a worthy, long-term ally.

THE 40 PERCENT SOLUTION?

There's other edible evidence that's at least as intriguing: "Eating more whole grains, vegetables and fruit may lower a person's risk for colorectal cancer by up to 40 percent," says research from the Fox Chase Cancer Center in Philadelphia. That stat is also cited in *The Cancer Prevention Diet* (St. Martin's Press), by Michio Kushi. Forty percent, I'd say, is too huge to ignore.

More than a mere quote, this citation serves to support the nutritional philosophies of "macrobiotic" diets, in which strict vegetarian, Asian-inspired, spartan eating plans have reportedly—and repeatedly—led to spontaneous healing among more than a few Stage IV cancer patients in the U.S. and Europe. The spontaneous, unexpected eradication of cancers may be more mystery than science at this point in the mid-2000s, but macrobiotic eating also makes sense for countless others who aren't patients or survivors (for more info, contact kushiinstitute.org). Despite the lack of steak-and-eggs breakfasts, the point is not to eat-to-stay-hungry...but that extremely healthful eating, without excess sugar, fat and calories, may help optimize the body's healing resources in ways that aren't yet fully understood.

One point proffered by Kushi, who subtitles his book: [the] *Nutritional Blueprint for the Prevention and Relief of Disease*, probably won't be displayed prominently in the halls of protein-powered, Atkins Diet doctors' offices. It reads: "Among the major forms of cancer, colon and breast cancer are now generally associated with a high-fat, high-protein diet by epidemiologists [who study disease]...."

I'VE SEEN FIRE AND I'VE SEEN RAW...

Before I sat down to write the first few-hundred words of this chapter, I hit the road in search of a futuristic, anti-cancer lunch. First stop: Pearl Street Mall, Boulder, Colorado, where I live, which is also the home of Celestial Seasonings Tea, the Herb Research Foundation, Olympic marathoner Frank Shorter ('72 and '76 Olympic champion), and the recently-licensed "fast-food" spot called Sally in the Raw.

Yes, there was a Sally; no, she wasn't nude. (That kind of establishment operates on the other side of town.) The Sally I met—who happens to be the tall, fit, engaging, curly-haired daughter of legendary singers James Taylor and Carly Simon—sold me a $6 portion of "pizza in the raw," which contained tomatoes, olives, sun-dried tomatoes, almonds, dates, garlic and lemon, on a buckwheat-and-sunflower seed crust...all of which was raised organically. More important: it was prepared like the rest of Sally in the Raw's food, at 110 degrees Fahrenheit or less. For in the New/Old World of "Raw" Cookery, chefs and devotees believe cooking with heat not only destroys many health benefits (including enzymes) of food; but that some foods cooked at high heat—for instance, red meat at over 300 degrees—create carcinogens, which can contribute to the development of cancer.

Sally and I didn't talk much about cancer, though. We talked instead about her health-inspired menu, and the freshness of it all; the variety; which also included a "mock" tuna-salad (almonds, sunflower seeds, celery, onion and kelp), plus "meatless loaf." All in all, a long way from crudités. Then, for another dollar, she served me a two-ounce drink, a shot of something called "Firewater." It looked like Hawaiian Punch-in-a-Nyquil cup but tasted like tepid Kool-Aid spiked with jalapeño pepper oil (turned out it was habañero). Sweet for a quick second, the firewater then promptly scorched my sinuses. Wasn't hardly sweet, but then Sally is selling longevity, not soda pop, out of the back of her tricked out '60s Volkswagen van/cart.

I felt properly healthy eating "raw," sitting in the sun, listening to a lunchtime bluegrass band, sipping fiery water…pondering the phytochemicals and other good stuff my nature-prepared pizza contained. I also pondered the fact that when Sally Taylor eats "raw," she says this kind of food makes her feel "tingly" all over. (Could be mere advertising hype, but a healthwise friend of mine who's tried it said much the same thing.) Still, I've got to say, I left the mall hungry. Which may, it turns out, contribute at least a little bit to nutri-aided longevity I may have gained since my cancer surgery a few years ago…. Sally & Co. don't advertise it, but eating raw means eating markedly fewer calories.

NEW PROTEIN "SHAKE" AGAINST NAUSEA?

As with humor, as with eating-during-chemo, "timing" can be everything. But a recent eye-opening study of a protein/ginger drink may well help untold thousands of cancer patients feel better during chemo—even perhaps reducing their need for (expensive) antiemetics (aka anti-vomit) pills. In short, researchers tested three groups of patients taking chemo (Journal of Alternative and Complementary Therapies, June. 1, 2008), and found that those who took high protein powder supplements, along with ginger, twice daily, fared markedly better than those who quaffed less protein, or no protein/ginger drinks at all. One tip noted in the small study: They started the "shakes" the day after chemo (timing!), when stomachs typically get worse. The docs stated: "High protein meals with ginger reduced the delayed nausea... and reduced use of [antiemetics]." Cheers to that.

UNDERNUTRITION WITHOUT MALNUTRITION

For cancer survivors and others interested in links between hunger and longevity, it may be time to set aside (temporarily) the leanings of popular, oft-times healthful, low-carb diets. And focus instead on nutrient-packed calories. Because whether it is "fair" or not, in terms of survival or living longer, eating fewer calories, for years on end—seems to mean more years of life than what experts might have previously predicted. I fully realize this sounds unfair at first, especially to people like me who have endured cancer, chemotherapy and surgery-related weight loss of 40 pounds or more. I mean: Is it fair to ask recovering patients to stay slightly hungry, for years on end? After all, these are people who were so sick for so long they could hardly eat, or keep from vomiting, for days....

But this is strict science talking, not a benevolent post-surgical psychotherapist. (For the record, I gained back 50 pounds eventually, after my surgery and treatment.) When all is said and done, compared and contrasted, the only way medical science consistently has shown to extend the lives of mammals in labs around the world since the 1950s, is to "underfeed" test mice, rabbits, dogs and, most recently (in U.S. government labs in Baltimore), chimpanzees. The goal of the research is "undernutrition without malnutrition," which means feeding subjects super-nutritious food, but in nutritious meals that don't quite fill the animals' stomachs. Ever. Pretty much without fail, it turns out, animals that have eaten extremely healthful meals, for months or years, have lived notably longer than their control counterparts, who were allowed to eat what they wished and when.

"With mice that are supposed to live 14 months," reported Dr. Kathleen Hall, speaking of the groundbreaking undernutrition studies run by the late Roy Walford, M.D., of the University of California, Los Angeles, some years ago, "he's got them living *four* years." That's a nearly 250 (!) percent increase in longevity, which is rather astounding, even if it's been achieved only in mice and not yet people.

This doesn't mean, though, that cancer survivors should ceaselessly go hungry, while following strict diets that feature only supernutritious foods. Nor should they try to "ape" the longer-living, hungry-by-design chimps that now dine daily at the National Institute on Aging labs in Baltimore. The point here is to simply state where the crossroads of calories and longevity-science meet. Then we as colon cancer survivors can pick and choose ways to try to simulate (within reason) the diets of animals that have outlived their predecessors (and scores of predictions). And if we choose to listen to the experts and crimp our cravings just slightly—and healthfully—for years or decades, many of us would likely benefit by leaning more toward the lean than the obese side of normal. Gotta say it again: This doesn't mean cancer survivors should diet-for-life. This hasn't yet been proven to work magic for humans. Nor is it much fun. The related science does, though, point to one metabolic fact: Most of the diet-related cancers in the world, including (many) colon cancers, tend to occur among those who are overfed, under-exercised, and not educated or practiced in medically-oriented eating.

"Sugar feeds cancer," says Patrick Quillin, Ph.D., and nutrition specialist, who wrote *Beating Cancer Through Nutrition*. Quillin also claims that malnutrition kills more than 40 percent of cancer patients. These are powerful statements that are difficult to ignore when planning to modify one's diet for the future, the long-term future.

LONGEVITY MENU #1

The menu below, adapted from the works of noted UCLA pathologist Roy Walford, M.D., is a one-day sample of how to eat for longevity, on a mere 1,500 calories or so. (Some research subjects who've tried the severe diet decided to eat a more normal amount of calories [1,700 to 2,000] for six days a week, then fast on the seventh.) When I interviewed Dr. Walford years ago (long before he died and well before he became a minor celebrity as a member of the *Survivor*-like Biosphere experiment in the '90s), I asked him if he didn't think that taking souped-up antioxidant vitamins and eating this way were "unnatural." His answer: "Cancer is natural." Here, then, his grub:

BREAKFAST

1 T. brewer's yeast in low-sodium tomato juice
2/3 cup rye cereal
3 T. wheat germ
1 T. wheat bran
1/2 cup strawberries
1.1/4 cup skim milk

LUNCH

2 sweet potatoes and 2 pears
2 cups spinach
1/2 cup buttermilk [yogurt]

DINNER

Skinless chicken
Lima bean salad
Any remaining potatoes and pears
1 cup green beans
1 cup grapefruit

[*Adapted from *How a Man Ages*, (Ballantine Books), by Curtis Pesmen and the editors of *Esquire*; and *Maximum Life Span* (W.W. Norton & Co.), by Roy Walford, M.D.]

LONGEVITY MENU #2

This menu sample, created well before the low-carbohydrate diet trend caught on in the U.S., is adapted from *The Cancer Recovery Eating Plan* (Times Books, NYC) by Daniel Nixon, M.D. with Jane A. Zanca. Maybe that's why the protein ; carbs; fats ratios break down as: 21% protein; 68% carbohydrate; 11% fats.

BREAKFAST

Total and All-Bran cereals, mixed, with skim milk and strawberries; orange; toast

SNACK A.M.

Apple

LUNCH

New England clam chowder; whole wheat bread; skim milk

SNACK P.M.

Fruit yogurt

DINNER

Black bean and cornmeal loaf (small portion, appetizer)
Chicken breast in tortilla sauce
Brown-rice pilaf
Jicama slaw
Warm apricot pudding

CHEESEBURGER IN PARADISE

"You ever get pissed at me that you ate healthy all those years, and I didn't?…" asks Geoff, on a rare day of candor-studded best-friend banter, "and you got cancer?" Truth is, I don't get ticked at Geoff for that: We've got different genes. And I actually worry about his health, now that I truly know how short life can be for far too many. And he is allowed to say stuff like this, we agree, because his mom died of cancer when he was 13 (and his dad, of diabetes complications three years later). Have another bacon-cheese, Pal-o-mine.

A SURVIVORS' FOOD PYRAMID (Part I)

In 2004, on assignment for *Esquire* magazine, I worked for a short while with John Briffa, a British doctor who specialized in nutrition and wrote the book, *Ultimate Health*. Our task: to replace the outdated U.S. Department of Agriculture food pyramid with something more healthful that adult men could use, time and again.

TOP Level (eat sparingly)

Cookies, muffins, bagels (white flour), white bread, refined sugar, potato chips

SECOND Level (in moderation)

Brown rice, sweet potatoes, white potatoes, whole grains, whole-wheat pastas, oats, yogurt, cold-pressed sunflower oil

THIRD Level

Buffalo, venison, lamb, grass-fed beef, chicken

BOTTOM Level (eat most often)

Fruits, vegetables, oily fish, beans, lentils, peas, nuts, seeds, olive oil

What I found most compelling about this eating plan, which isn't quite a diet, is that it is based on an evolutionary philosophy, not a fad. It's closer to the Paleo (as in Paleolithic Man, how he ate, way back when) Diet than the Atkins and other low-carbohydrate plans, but the science behind it says we should eat closer to the ways we did in the wild. Fact is, we've eaten meat, vegetables, fish, for 200,000 or so years, but trans-fatty foods for fewer than 100 years. Guess which we're better at using—and digesting—over time?

A SURVIVORS' PYRAMID (Part II)

If only colon cancer were about one thing. Cheeseburgers. Broccoli. Or candy bars for chrissakes. But anybody who's been through one course of diagnosis/surgery/treatment knows better. At some point we realize our nutritional goals have changed: They now aim more toward immune-boosting intake than merely gaining weight post-op, or searching for the best, seared wild salmon available at any restaurant-of-the-moment.

When I approached the staff at the Jay Monahan Center for Gastrointestinal Health, a division of New York-Presbyterian Hospital/ Cornell Medical School, in search of a better food pyramid for colorectal cancer survivors and patients, they did two things. They handed me a book, *What Your Doctor May Not Tell You About Colorectal Cancer*, written by Mark Bennett Pochapin, M.D., director of the center, and steered me to Lynn Goldstein, an effervescent, knowledgeable dietitian who spends hours, days, months each year, figuring out exactly what's best to send down the gullets of those suffering from digestive diseases.

Dr. Pochapin, not unlike Dr. Nixon at the top of this chapter, believes there's protective benefit offered by healthful foods and supplements. He's cautious in his dietary pronouncements ("While I do believe in supplementation, I do not believe… there is a single magical agent that can prevent cancer.") Yet Pochapin also says later in the book, without hesitation, that the following five agents show "some promise in preventing colorectal cancer:"

1) Folic acid
2) Calcium
3) Vitamin D
4) Selenium
5) Vitamin E

For her part, in focusing more on nutrient-dense foods than supplements, dietitian Goldstein agrees with Pochapin and adds some unlikely meal choices in assembling a pyramid to help sustain long-term cancer survivors.

THE COLON CANCER SURVIVORS' FOOD PYRAMID

TOP LEVEL - 10%

Healthy fats (unsaturated, non-trans-fat oils, i.e. "Smart Balance" margarine substitute)

MID-LEVEL - 30%

Lean protein, fish , organic turkey; avoid long-cooked red meat

BOTTOM LEVEL - 60%

Plant-based foods, including vegetables, grains, legumes and nuts

The pyramid for colon cancer survivors (if there were such a U.S.-sanctioned federal tool) would have, as its base, 60 percent plant-based foods (fruits, vegetables, whole grains, legumes, nuts, seeds), according to Goldstein. The middle level, consisting of approximately 30 percent of the pyramid, comprises lean protein choices. At the top of the pyramid lies another 10 percent of one's (allowed) daily calories, in the form of so-called "healthy" fats: olive oil and unsaturated sunflower oil, to name two. By all accounts, it's wise to limit or reduce the amount of trans-fatty acids, which usually are found on the label under the heading "partially hydrogenated. "And don't forget water," Goldstein advises. "Your body is 60 percent water. You need at least two liters each day of non-caffeinated, non-sugared soft drink or similar."

Folate, Folic Acid, For Life

When it's in food, it's folate. When it's in a vitamin supplement, it's folic acid. Either way, getting a 400 to 1,000 micrograms of folate (a B vitamin) into your bloodstream each day is a wise way to help build a biochemical defense against polyps growing in the colon or colorectal cancer recurrence. Be mindful, though: A daily dose of more than 1,000 mg can be problematic for some patients, as folic acid can interfere with chemotherapy drugs, as well as mask deficiencies of Vitamin B12. Some top foods for folate include:

FOOD	FOLIC ACID/ amount mcg per serving
Asparagus	243
Black Beans	256
Broccoli	168
Lentils	358
Orange juice, concentrate	109
Orange juice, raw	74
Rice, long grain, enriched	797
Soup, minestrone, with water	51
Spinach	263
Taco Salad (fast food)	113
Turkey	485

WHEAT GERM: FOOD OR ANTI-CANCER MED?

When I first noticed the suggestion of wheat germ for longevity (see Longevity Diet, p. 138), I didn't give it much thought. But that was then. Now I, and a legion of others, do give it more thought. For in 2003, the *British Journal of Cancer* reported that wheat germ extract (also known as WGE, and Avemar in Europe), can help colorectal cancer patients' recovery, and may even have anti-tumor effects.

True, as with many studies of nutrition-and-cancer, the experimental population here was small (clinical trials can cost $millions; foods and herbs usually can't "pay back" the investors and makers nearly as quickly as Big Pharmaceutical-made drugs). But I also found that Memorial Sloan-Kettering, one of the world's leading cancer hospitals, found room on its Website to say, at least in modest support, that: "WGE is used as a dietary supplement by cancer patients in Hungary to improve quality of life," and also that: "Data from pilot studies [shows] a beneficial role for WGE in patients with colorectal cancer." This all tells me it's worth asking my/your "onc" about.

CHAPTER 7

Intimate Matters: Bedroom, Bathroom, Beyond

You hear a lot of medi-speak as a cancer patient. Too much, in fact. You forget a lot of it, too; your ears glaze over. Call it another coping mechanism. Yet there's one quote I haven't forgotten, nearly four years since a doctor spoke it. When I first heard those words, less than a month after diagnosis, I knew I had to write it down because it said something bizarre, and urgent, about the world I had unwillingly entered:

EIGHT WORDS YOU DON'T WANT TO HEAR

"There I am, below ground, splayed out on a hard exam table in the UCSF radiation-therapy room, hospital-pajama bottoms pulled halfway down my crotch...when a senior member of the radiation/oncology team addresses a younger doctor after

" How apart we feel now... "

– Jill G., 40, wife of colon cancer patient now in remission viewing my simulation—the precise position I will be in when radiation beams will enter my body. He uses eight words: 'The penis is going to have a reaction.' In other words, the penis (which would be mine) will very likely develop a severe sunburn of sorts, over six weeks of absorbing adjacent, anti-cancer radiation waves. Note to self: 'Prepare.' "

BEDROOM NOTES:

THE POWER OF TOUCH

What I didn't want, despite all the kind offers sent my way, was anybody to touch me after my surgery; after being prepped, poked, anal-probed, radiated, carved, re-routed, stapled together, benumbed, and finally, wheelchair-discharged. What I didn't want was anybody to touch me…including, at times, my wife. Not a healthful situation, it would seem, after all she had done for me over six, seven, nine months' time.

Point is, I remember thinking this at first while Paula was having a "housecall" massage, soon after her scoliosis-addled back reared up and brought her down. I wasn't envious of the soothing, oil-infused, tender care she was receiving in the room next door. Nor was I jealous that the massage therapist was a guy. (Alright, maybe a touch jealous of that.) I simply knew I'd rather be all by my lonesome, near-wretching with chemo-nausea…staring at a tepid bowl of macaroni and cheddar while watching ESPN baseball…than having some soft-talking masseuse pressing in on my body with his scrubbed-pink, über-trained fingertips and thumbs…digging all in and his palms providing punctuation. Me? I was just fine 15 feet from him—feeling post-traumatic-heck-with-em. I was living largely horizontal, in a state 40 pounds lighter than when I started this treatment gig. Point is, as the able-bodied fans stood up and took a seventh-inning stretch on TV, I improvised and rolled over onto my side. And wondered whether I was building a shell of sorts around me.

THE POWER OF GYNECOLOGICAL TOUCH

In spring, 2001, William Fuller, M.D., then-chairman of Obstetrics and Gynecology at Health One's Presbyterian-St. Luke's Hospital in Denver, who's delivered more than 5,000 babies in over 20 years of practice, pulls me aside and tells me that, because of the stories I've written about my cancer and my misdiagnosis, he is changing how he practices medicine. He will now add digital (rectal) exams to the standard workup in his patients' checkups if they are over age 40 or at risk for colorectal cancer. For many women, these digital exams had been optional—they simply weren't thought of as automatic Ob-Gyn terrain. This means, in part, the publicity of my case will help, if not immediately save lives, then at least improve the future sex lives of an untold number of Dr. Fuller's patients—and those of their partners.

THE POWER OF TUMESCENCE

When you're fighting for your life, it's not surprising to find the importance of orgasm isn't, well, as important as it was before. That's not to say sex isn't important; it's more a sad fact of survivor reality.

In my case, after hearing from three different doctors that I may lose some or all of my "powers of erection" after tricky colorectal surgery that would take place in part near my prostate gland, I remember feeling, with my wife at my side, both embarrassed and resigned: "Okay...then..., maybe it's Viagra for life." With an emphasis on "for life."

It's a deal I was prepared to make, to exit my surgery cancer-free. (It's also not as if I had a bushel of options.) In order to excise a large, Stage III tumor embedded in and around the rectum, the surgeons at University of California-San Francisco's Moffitt Hospital were going to have to be both aggressive and unusually sensitive—sensitive, that is, to all sorts of nerves bundled near my prostate and perineum (beneath the sub-dermal section from scrotum to anus) that have lots to do with how erections form…and perform. (For women, Ob-Gyns have informed me, orgasmic waves happen here….)

Looking back, I'd never call myself "lucky" after what I'd faced at a relatively young age—43—and after enduring a missed diagnosis or three. But I consider myself extremely fortunate in one regard: Thanks to the profuse skill (plus experimental, nerve-tracking, nerve-sparing technique) of surgeons Welton and Carroll, I can forthrightly report that at 46, I've yet to require the "oomph" services of such esteemed pharmaceuticals as Levitra, Viagra or Cialis. The docs got my cancer out, and in expertly doing so saved my innate powers of…tumescence.

SEX AND MY CANCER (Part I)

Early on in my treatment, I had a mini-confessional:

"Haven't yet poked around the standard patient Web sites about sex and colon cancer…," I reported. "Here's what I know so far: In one month of being a colon-cancer patient, I've had sex twice; once what I would term successfully. The other time, well, that's what I know about sex and my cancer."

AM I NORMAL, YET?

When is sex not quite sex? One answer, according to Terry Real, Ph.D., a marital and family therapist in Cambridge, Massachusetts, and author of *The New Rules of Marriage,* is: when people are feeling undue pressures about major life events. These pressures, which arise during financial upheavals and recovery from such major illnesses as heart attack and cancer, can lead to unexpected and uncomfortable moments in bed. Even between eager, compatible sex partners.

"His nerves may cause him to seek sex when all he really wants is reassurance or some support from his partner," Real explained to me. "It's just that he might find it easier to reach out for that support under the covers late at night rather than in the kitchen, face-to-face…. He may want to talk, but what he knows to do is grab her in bed."

Guilty as charged. This was, at times, undeniably true in my case, and, I'm guessing, in countless others'. We may not often say it, but I will here: As mind/body-damaged survivors, we may want so badly to prove we're back to "normal," that we can hardly help using sex as a crutch. Makes it difficult, then, for maybe the first six months to a year post-op, to consider sex a playful event. Which is not to say we shouldn't have it. Or enjoy it. Real and his therapist colleagues aren't preaching that: They are looking instead to lead us to acknowledging weighty feelings of inadequacy and (possibly misplaced) fears of mortality. Then, it's hoped, we can finally relax into sex once again.

SEX AND MY CANCER (Part II)

Less than two months after diagnosis you could say I was tired; you could also say I was fried:

"Wondering, in bed, how long it will take for the barbecued, irradiated skin on my package to return to normal color and texture…. Finding that having an erection and doing something pleasurable with it hurts in such odd, frightening ways in the first weeks after radiation treatment…that it makes you think twice about having an erection and doing something pleasurable with it."

SEXOLOGICAL, ONCOLOGICAL GYNECOLOGY

Back before cancer put a crimp in my sex life, I discovered one "hot" new way to have better sex: What happened was, *Glamour* magazine hired me to write an article about new "lust lotions" women were trying out (under doctor supervision), to see if Viagra-type drugs, or creams, might work for them. Nice work.

The theory was similar to how men's erection drugs work, except that the lotions would be applied by hand, not popped in pill form. The goal: to boost blood flow to the vagina and clitoris in order to increase female sexual arousal or orgasms. One company, Vivus, even received a patent for such a specific, hormone-based cream. In researching these drugs, I learned a key lesson in female anatomy: the clitoris, like the penis, is much larger than it may at first appear. In fact the primary female sex organ contains countless bundles of nerves, arteries, veins and capillaries—a whole network of potential for pleasure. These nerves and vessels run beneath the clitoral (or erectile) shaft and spread both inward, toward the rectum, and outward, toward the thighs. Instead of a mere "pea-shaped organ," then, the clitoris can be described (depending upon the gynecologist doing the describing) as a longer, stronger, "inverted Y-shaped organ," in which the tongs of the "Y," or the pea-pods if you will, reach into the groin, well beyond the vagina.

The reason I'm recalling all this now is because I received a recent e-mail from a fellow-colon cancer survivor who happened to be female. And whose surgery happened to have some unfortunate Ob-Gyn complications:

"I'm trying to be active," Laurie B. said. "I can't do walking very well, as the radiation gave me second- and third-degree burns. I have had to accept a new normal.... And because of my treatments, as soon as I put food in my mouth I have to find the bathroom....

"That's just part of it," she added. "But I've been lucky. I had a three-year colonoscopy last week; it was clean, NED [no evidence of disease]. But life changes and there I am, four days later [with], orangutan bottom. When I walk too far, it goes to bleeding.

"The radiation took away all the soft tissue," Laurie explained, comparing her rectal cancer treatment to mine. [Except that her surgical side effects seemed to affect some spinal nerves as well; and are more feminine.] "I have to be dilated, because the rectum-to-sphincter [tissue] tries to shrink. It's like sitting on an open sore. I was also damaged vaginally: The gynecologist has to use a pediatric instrument to examine me. I had a reversal (of a stoma) on September 10, 2001; now they want to put the colostomy back on."

And I was worried, not too long ago, about a possible future need to simply swallow some Cialis for better sex.

TRICK FAQ?

A story in *GQ* magazine—arguably the modern metrosexual man's embodiment of fashion and style in print—once asked a simple question: "What is a man's most powerful sex organ? The answer is the brain."

It went on: "What, then, is a man's second most powerful sex organ? The answer is the skin."

Point is, skipping the technicalities: No matter what happens, temporarily or more permanently, to a cancer patient's crotch—as a result of chemotherapy, radiation or surgery—there's a lot left to play with; a lot left to enjoy.

SEX AND MY CANCER [Part III]

So there I am, a few weeks after surgery—more than three, but who's counting?—I'm fooling around in bed with Paula, and it feels like high school fooling-around-in-bed....Because, honestly, I don't know what will happen...on my side of the bed...if we keep this up. Fact is...plumbing's been shut off for a while. Lotsa hands, more than usual, it seems. And I'm not thinking about baseball or the Queen Mother. I'm thinking, for a few seconds at least, about the doctor who warned me that I might be Viagra-dependent...for a while. For a long while.

Maybe for decades...but...not...now...."First time since surgery," I'm thinking, feeling a lot like in high school right now, with lotsa hands...and an odd, resurgent, genital-tickle-toward-inevitability...and a rhythmic pumping in the erection that almost wasn't...hold on...on the verge...of bringing unfamiliar groans of pleasure.

Feels so good I feel like shouting but I don't. Instead I'll just write about it, quietly, in the pages of a nationally published book. And maybe take a nap.

BATHROOM NOTES:

A FRIEND WANTS TO KNOW...

"Do you think about cancer every day?" a friend writes, a friend who doesn't really know my whole story, but who wants to know more.

"Yes," I answer, "in part because they took out my colon during surgery...." (Hope I didn't sound angry when answering him, 'cause it's been five or six months since the operation.) "Yes," in other words, because I now have a handicap. "Yes," because I'm now what the gastro-cancer health professionals call, an "ostomate." There's colostomy, where the colon gets re-routed through the torso; and ileostomy, where the small intestine is what's left. That's me. Not a major handicap, some would say—compared with the likes of Stephen Hawking or what Christopher Reeve endured. But as one of the vast minority (approximately 15 percent) of colorectal cancer patients who sacrificed a bowel or rectum in order to become cancer-free, I can't help but think about cancer two, three, maybe four brief times a day—when I have to use the bathroom in an unconventional way; when I empty the contents of my polyethylene pouch into the toilet, before flushing, before washing my hands (like everybody else), and before going back on the other side of the bathroom door...into the world where I won't think about cancer, least for a while.

CAN ABS BE TOO STRONG?

They didn't warn my cancer-stricken pal beforehand. Maybe because they didn't know. When young Martin (not his real name), all of 35, found out he was slated to have a temporary ileostomy diverted through his lower torso during rectal cancer surgery, he did a smart thing. He took some time and tried to get into shape for the operation. Rowing machine, swimming, ab work: the guy did his homework.

Problem was, after the surgery (successful!) to remove his cancer, his stoma didn't function properly. In fact it hardly functioned at all. No light through the end of the tunnel. Which caused him extreme, lose-major-sleep pain and misery, as all sorts of undue pressure was being exerted on a section of small intestine that was not working. For unknown reasons (including possible surgical error), it was not allowing food to pass out of the body, through the temporary and new-fashioned anus, while the rest of his digestive tract healed. They said it might take six-to-eight weeks. Trouble was, Martin had abs. Honest-to-goodness abs, bordering on six-pack; earned from years of sustained, teeth-clenching ab exercises. And yet, unfortunately for him, the muscularity of the six-pack seemingly bunched up around the detoured small intestine and apparently pinched it shut, like a crimp in a garden hose you left out all winter. (His ileostomy, like most, was threaded through the ab muscles and out the lower torso.) Next time, he and his family vowed—though they hope to heavens they'll never see a next time—he'll let himself get a bit more squidgy in and around the middle. For "health" reasons; just to be safe.

THE RESECTION: THE HEALING COLON

Most people who have colon cancer, it bears repeating, don't end up with a permanent colostomy. In truth, fewer than 20 percent face this type of digestive-disease-related disfigurement. In the hospital there's a cutting out of diseased colon, maybe 6 inches, maybe a foot and a half (of the total five to six feet) or more (in my case the whole organ). Then comes "resection," which means stitching together of the two remaining sections that have been rendered "open" during the surgery. In general, in approximately 20 percent of colon cancer surgeries, the patient's bowel habits are noticeably and at times frustratingly affected.

In the best case scenario…resection that is done during first surgery…all intestines wake up and start working within 24-to-48 hours. A clean resection. But with cancer, as we've seen, things don't always go cleanly. Depending upon which portion(s) of the colon were removed, patients often have to adjust to a new schedule of bowel movements, replete with new habits.

Sometimes survivors will heal on schedule, yet never feel as if their bowels are quite emptied. Other times frequency (three times a day instead of one) or consistency of stools change markedly. (With less colon in place, there's less organ tissue with which to remove water from your waste.) There's no doubt a nurse will review all this with you—if she or he hasn't already—before your discharge from the hospital. You may even be warned that you'll need to "retrain yourself" a bit on going to the toilet. But it's a tough thing to talk about—taking a dump, anew. It's a tough thing to even want to talk about.

THE SYMPTOMS, SECOND TIME AROUND

Most of us know the Big Five, the warning signs of colorectal cancer: 1] abdominal cramping; 2] blood in the stool or toilet; 3] rectal bleeding; 4] thinning stools; and 5] "false" urges to have a bowel movement. But we also know early stage colon cancer may be masked by other conditions (constipation, inflammatory bowel disease). So, besides tracking your CEA (carcinoembryonic antigen) test two or three times per year, anyone especially concerned about recurrence may want to talk with their oncologist about using at-home stool or fecal-occult blood tests.

The tests are portable, private, and now over-the-counter. They also inadvertently turn your toilet into a forensic device, as you hunt "invisible" intestinal blood in the privacy of your bathroom. By simply taking a smear of stool from tissue (using a gloved hand if you prefer) and sending the wrapped plastic swab-utensils to the lab, survivors can rather easily add an extra layer of prevention and assurance to their year-round, anti-cancer efforts. There are even newer, more high-tech tests, such as those made by the Exact Sciences Corporation, which use genetic markers to screen bowel movements for early signs of colorectal cancer. Big plus: the specimen "collections" are made in the privacy of your own home. (for more information, check: Exactsciences.com)

THE ENDORSEMENT: THE BAG

It is not exactly pretty; it is something I am not exactly proud of. The bag I now wear, along with thousands of other colorectal-cancer survivors, is a flesh-colored, polyethylene utensil not that different in shape or appearance from a flattened, up side-down, old-fashioned milk bottle, the kind you see at carnivals and county fairs—"Three throws for a dollar...knock 'em off the table!"

The bag is two fists tall or thereabouts, reaching, as I stand, from next to my navel to the glans of my (nonerect) penis. The bag, also called "the pouch" by ostomy experts, is emptied three times a day and at bedtime and changed every three days or so. Featuring two openings—one that attaches to my lower torso with skin-friendly adhesives, the other that empties into the toilet and clips shut—the bag is a lot better alternative than an adult diaper, I'd say; others might say, cynically, "That Depends." I would not however say that. For the bag is hidden under boxers and is airtight-watertight-hygienic. Even as it is not exactly attractive.

THE NON-ENDORSEMENT: THE BAG

Accidents will happen. In the notable, 1997 nonfiction book *Man-to-Man*, author and publishing exec Michael Korda talks about how, leading up to his diagnosis of prostate cancer, he dealt with the fact that his urogenital works—bladder/prostate/penis—were in trouble. He knew this in part because he had started charting particular pedestrian pathways—en route to his office everyday—through and around parking lots in Midtown Manhattan, so he could easily reach the rare, open-to-public bathrooms, before his bladder gave out from urgency and inflammation. He was a 60-year-old man who felt older.

In my case, my ostomy bags have leaked five or six times over nearly four years. Twice, minor leaks followed extended airplane trips, coincidentally or not (maybe the cabin pressure?). Two more times bags have pulled partly away following unexpected athletic-type moves (not on playing fields or golf courses, but in an office and outside next to a parking lot). They've more admirably survived ski mountain falls, swimming pools, hot tubs (though not recommended for long stretches of time), twice-weekly mountain bike rides, a 10-K road race at altitude, and an untold number of a two-year-old's climbing-on-Daddy maneuvers. Sure, stuff happens. But there's usually an early warning, a tension signal-on-skin that signals the wearer to head to the john for repairs. And it doesn't happen nearly as frequently as I, or my fellow "ostomates," would have thought (www.uoaa.org or see Appendix II).

WISE WORDS: LESSONS FROM THE
SURGICAL WARD FRONT LINES

After 20 years of caring for colorectal cancer patients, most of whom have had major surgery, Susan Barbour, R.N., of the University of California-San Francisco, is a human website/encyclopedia of sorts when it comes to a survivor's most personal feelings. She counseled me before and after my surgery, taught me how to live with an ileostomy; and somehow I felt we would always share a strong, if odd, connection. Sure enough, when I contacted her to help with this chapter, it felt as if we'd only been "apart" for a few months. Life-saving surgery does have a way of bringing people...closer.

"Ostomy issues are so loaded in our society," she says. "If the child, spouse or friend of a patient has issues with it, those issues come through to the patient. If you're uncomfortable with it, it comes through. I'll often ask the spouse direct questions if I have a feeling [there's discomfort there]. We go talk in the hallway; I try to normalize it."

Regarding the bathroom inevitables, Barbour says, "Gloves—people ask if they should wear gloves to change the bag. I say, 'Do you wear gloves when you go? When you change a baby's diaper?' It's kind of the same thing. That's something everybody asks, gloves. I downplay that. I'm a minimalist. Some nurses come in with a suitcase full of supplies, gizmos.

"Sometimes family members want to do a lot, to help, change it. I say, okay, but I find out what the patient wants. I force the issue—I make sure the partner sees it in the hospital, in a supportive environment. I'll show the stoma to them. One woman thought her stoma was temporary, so she put off intimacy with her husband—she didn't want him to see it. It turned out, after a year and a half, to be a permanent stoma. They had no sex for a year and a half. Another couple, I had a lesbian couple, they were in their 60s: The patient was concerned with the stoma; that her partner wouldn't like her as much. I tell them the patient needs to believe the partner when

157

they say, 'I love you and don't care.' I'd say 90 percent (of partners) don't care…. But some people get compulsive with it."

In rapid-fire succession, nurse Barbour shared a handful of other insights, providing answers to colorectal questions I didn't know I had: "Some of the right things to say, to patients after surgery are: 'How are you doing? You look terrific.' When it comes to farts [in which gas from the small intestine rushes into the bag, briefly, instead of out of the usual orifice], I tell patients/partners to acknowledge them. Humor helps make light. 'Your stoma's talking to me….' It's worse to ignore them.

"As for intimacy, the partner often feels like they will hurt them. It's up to me to let them know they won't. Some people are terrified of hurting the patient, from just hugging, or anything physical. I had this [one] couple, in which stomach stroking was part of their routine. It was integrated into their foreplay. The partner was asking what to do? I said, 'Move along; you have the whole other side.'

"I might push people sometimes to get together, to talk and learn about the stoma [stuff]. Some people think it's temporary, but you never know when it's over. You don't want to let a piece of intestine on the outside get between them."

Personal Questions – and Answers

Of all that's wrong with the internet, one of the things that's right about it is how quickly it can offer—and deliver—answers to some of the most personal questions a person might have. Including questions of medically-affected sex, reproduction, elimination (as in the other kind of toiletry) and communication (as in therapy, psycho- or marital). Here are four top-notch places to turn when you don't quite have the right person available, right there next to you, to answer a few, or more, questions of urgency. Rest assured: These folks have Heard it All Before.

1. American Association for Marital and Family Therapy (AAMFT)
Alexandria, VA (703) 838-9808

In 20-plus years of practicing medical journalism, I've attended dozens if not hundreds of seminars, conferences and press conferences at which doctors or other health professionals have gathered to find or pitch solutions to our mind/body ills. I've also found, over the years, that the AAMFT annual meetings offer incredibly sound, practical, helpful advice to patients, clients, and couples in need of short- or long-term therapy (even when they aren't aware they need therapy). Though the annual meetings aren't open to the public, the AAMFT website is. It can help match therapists and clients nationwide, in a snap. www.AAMFT.org

2. National Coalition for Cancer Survivorship (NCCS)
Silver Spring, MD (877) 622-7937 (toll-free) www.canceradvocacy.org

After the surgery, after the treatment, after all the hands-on help, here's a safe, scientifically-sound place to go to connect with those interested in guiding you through the next phase of healing. Particularly helpful when you're more alone than you're used to being (and when your caregiver, perhaps, needs a little time off).

159

3. United Ostomy Association (UOA)

Irvine, CA (800) 826-0826 www.uoaa.org

This group, and its invaluable chat-lines, comprising specialized nurses, doctors, therapists and online patient advocates, tells it absolutely Like It Is. A major source of stress-relief to those who are dealing with colostomy, ileostomy or urostomy (urological stomas) issues for the first, or follow-up, times.

4. *Intimate Partners* by Maggie Scarf (Ballantine Books, 1988)

No website needed, no doctors, no nurses, no cancer focus. Merely the best book I've ever read about getting closer to someone you love. It also offers staggeringly clear reasons why it is so difficult for husband and wife, boyfriend-girlfriend, or partner and partner, to connect at the highest, most significant, levels. It's got sex, psychology, infidelity, plus case studies. Bonus: Written by a writer, not a psychotherapist.

www.randomhouse.com or online booksellers such as bn.com.

CHAPTER 8

Back to the Office: Job Tips, Insurance Solutions

Not unlike most cancer activists, Barbara Hoffman got involved because a loved one suffered through the disease: herself. As a 19-year-old Hoffman was diagnosed with Hodgkin's. She clung to her goal of becoming a lawyer, though vowing at an idealistic age to help people with illness and disability. Her adversity was our gain. These days, Hoffman is one of America's leading authorities and activists on the employment rights of cancer survivors.

In a few key ways, cancer survivors' quality-of-life has improved on the job since the Americans with Disabilities Act or ADA became law in the early 1990s. (Not nearly as much as Hoffman and many of us would like, mind you, but it's gotten better.) One main reason is employers are more aware that

" The biggest role the Americans with Disabilities Act plays for cancer survivors going back to work is it discourages discrimination in the first place. "

– Barbara Hoffman, general counsel, National Coalition for Cancer Survivorship people diagnosed with cancer do return to productive careers in the work-force. Another factor: Our size. There are about 10 million cancer sur-vivors in the U.S. today. Roughly half plan to return to jobs and careers or, in the case of childhood cancers, start them. We are far less likely, than a generation ago, to be denied the very normal job and health insurance portions of the very normal lives all cancer survivors desire.

THAT'S THE GOOD NEWS...

"We have successfully persuaded most everyone to use the word 'sur-vivor' instead of 'victim,' " says Hoffman, a professor of law at Rutgers University in New Jersey. "The ADA has helped changed those percep-tions." Laws have a way of doing that. So does that fact that virtually everyone knows a friend or family member who has overcome cancer. We see examples of normal, productive lives led by cancer survivors every day.

But, and there's always a "but" when you're talking jobs or insurance, cases such as these "overheard" on the National Cancer Institute's (NCI) colorectal cancer chat lines (www.cancer.gov) are still more here-and-now than anyone would want to admit. "After I had my colostomy, my employer asked me to quit my job because the cancer was upsetting my fellow workers," said survivor/patient Jon H. "He said a demotion or transfer was possible if I didn't agree. Except for my wife, that job was my whole world. So rather than quit, I decided to fight for it."

In a slightly different vein, survivor Roy P., recalls, "When I went back to work, my boss was honest with me. She said that my situation had been discussed at a managers' meeting. Some people had questioned what impact my coming back would have on the company's insurance rates. Her boss asked how she planned to get the job done with an employee (me) she could no longer 'count on' to stay healthy. Fortunately, she did some research and found out that the turnover rate, absenteeism records and work performance of people with a cancer history are very much the same as unaffected workers. Her facts helped correct management's wrong ideas."

When a survivor has been wronged by an employer or insurance carrier, one area in which the ADA falls short is in effecting a clear remedy. Court decisions vary widely and there is continued hot debate about whether cancer (overall or by specific type) even qualifies as a disability under the Act. "Lawsuits don't always get the results you want and they cost money," says Hoffman. These are two solid reasons why any cancer survivor needs to be proactive about the vital issues of health insurance and job rights. (And remember: Disability coverage varies by insurer—some require you "use up" all your sick and family leave first.)

GETTING YOUR JOB BACK, OR A NEW ONE

In total, forty percent of people diagnosed with cancer are adults in the work force. They want to go back to their jobs and careers after treatment. Four out of five indeed do return to work, while research shows cancer survivors are no less productive or absent from work than other co-workers. Straightforward talk with your employer, especially your supervisors and key co-workers, is the best way to disarm any notion that you can't return to the workforce or the job you held before treatment. One point to make clear is the treatment period is naturally going to be more challenging than the months and years that follow once you've put cancer behind you.

The federal Family and Medical Leave Act can be an ally. It requires employers with 50 or more employees to provide up to 12 weeks of unpaid but job-protected leave to address your own serious illness. It also requires employers to continue to provide health insurance and other benefits during the leave period, plus give back your position or its equivalent when you return.

163

Then, too, there are provisions to govern both employees (such as making reasonable efforts to schedule treatments to minimize workplace disruptions or loss of productivity) and employers (allowing an intermittent or reduced work schedule when "medically necessary"). The Family and Medical Leave Act, along with the ADA, make up part of a core of laws you'll want to get comfortable with, at least in broad strokes, as you refashion your life as a survivor.

For starters, you may ask, "How do I get health insurance with this now pre-existing condition of cancer? How will employers look at my resumé with the gap of professional experience that matches up with surgery and other treatments? How should I respond to questions about my health?" The National Coalition of Cancer Survivorship or NCCS makes these cogent recommendations for reducing "the chance of discrimination" when seeking a new job:

- Do not volunteer that you have or have had cancer unless it directly affects your qualifications for the job. Don't ask about health insurance until after receiving a job offer and only then ask about the "benefits package."

- Do not lie on the job or insurance application. If you are hired and your employer later learns that you lied, you may be fired. Or insurance may refuse to pay benefits and/or cancel coverage.

- If possible, seek positions with larger employers. Hoffman, for one, believes they are less likely to discriminate or be misinformed than smaller companies.

- Keep in mind your legal rights. The ADA stipulates an employer cannot (legally) ask about your medical history or request medical records before making a conditional job offer. If there is a conditional offer, the employer can ask for medical records or an exam only if it is required of all job applicants.

- Keep the focus on your current ability to do the job. The Office of Survivorship (a relatively new division) at the National Cancer Institute recommends practicing possible answers to health history questions before any interview. Be confident and avoid sounding defensive. If you have to explain an extended work absence, do it in a way that shows your illness decidedly in the past tense. Hoffman recommends substituting the name of your exact cancer ("lymphoma" or "adenocarcinoma") to avoid using a word that still carries myth and misperception. It is a wise move to have a note from your doctor on medical center stationery to vouch for your ability to perform job duties. Plus, it should reflect your current good/competent health status and the expectation you will likely have normal longevity. The NCI suggests working with a career or jobs counselor to put your best foot—and health outlook—forward.

One oft-overlooked point: "Don't discriminate against yourself by assuming you have a disability," says Hoffman. She urges survivors to make an honest assessment of work-life capabilities—then develop a targeted job search to reflect the assessment.

Pre-existing Condition Questions

When you first join a group health plan—either after finding a new job or as a cancer survivor (or both)—you'll likely be asked about your medical history. What to do? Or when you make a claim during the first year of coverage, the insurance carrier can check to see if you received drugs or other treatment that would indicate a preexisting condition. If so, the insurance carrier might apply its "preexisting condition exclusion," and deny coverage or reimbursement for up to a year.

Having a preexisting condition, however, such as "cancer two years ago," does not mean you will not be covered. It depends on your plan, as well as the timing. Importantly, a condition is defined as "preexisting" only if diagnosis, medical advice, care or treatment was actually received or recommended during the six-month period ending on the date you enrolled in the group health plan. This means if you're a cancer survivor who doesn't require any special follow-up care or monitoring, no preexisting-condition waiting period can (legally) be administered.

FROM SURVIVOR TO "INSURED SURVIVOR"

Aside from the formidable physical damage described elsewhere in these pages, cancer wreaks financial havoc as well. For instance, losing a job—or not quite focusing on it while fighting to regain your health—brings the additional collateral damage of jeopardizing your health insurance coverage. Especially if, as with most Americans, you are tied at least partly to a group health insurance plan.

Here, cobbled by experts, is a short course on what you need to know about keeping or obtaining health insurance after cancer. For more tips and details, consult the Resources box for new developments. One other key move: Request the latest revised (that's important) copy of "What

Cancer Survivors Need to Know about Health Insurance" from the National Coalition for Cancer Survivorship (NCCS) and make it your unofficial bible for insurance matters (www.canceradvocacy.org). Karen Pollitz, one of the co-authors of the NCCS booklet, routinely speaks to cancer survivor groups for 45 minutes to an hour on this exact topic. Her most important advice?

"Your protections [to keep or find health insurance] depend on where you live, very much where you live," says Pollitz, project director of the Institute for Health Care Research and Policy at Georgetown University. Heading into 2005, five states have decreed all residents be guaranteed individual health insurance, no matter the circumstances: New York, New Jersey, Maine, Vermont and Massachusetts. There are four other states, plus Washington D.C., in which Blue Cross/Blue Shield must sell you an individual policy: Michigan, Pennsylvania, Virginia and North Carolina.

THE TWO MUST-KNOW LAWS

On a national scale, two laws known as COBRA and HIPAA serve as allies for cancer survivors. They provide protection in many cases, but it is vital to know how and when these laws apply in your individual state. COBRA (Consolidated Omnibus Budget Reconciliation Act) requires employers to offer group medical coverage to employees and dependents who otherwise would lose group coverage by quitting, getting fired or having their working hours reduced. The national law requires COBRA insurance to be offered by any company with 20 or more employees. Some states have "mini-COBRA" laws that require the same of small companies with fewer than 20 workers.

COBRA basically "buys" you time to enroll in another health insurance plan, though you have to pay your former employer's part of the premium. You are allowed 18 months of COBRA coverage to make the transition to another health plan.

HIPAA, also known at the Kassebaum-Kennedy Act, is intended to help individuals with serious health conditions by removing past barriers (such as turning down a person with preexisting conditions) when trying to get health insurance or keep it when changing jobs. Specifically, HIPAA requires "nondiscrimination" among group health plans. That means group health plans cannot single out cancer survivors because of health status in order to deny, limit or charge more for health coverage.

Note that this is how HIPAA works for groups. If you need to buy individual health insurance, once again it matters greatly where you live. In some states, insurers can deny coverage, charge higher premiums or refuse to cover any preexisting condition. Other states, as mentioned, have fixed this injustice. But you will still pay higher premiums because it is an individual plan that doesn't afford the economies of scale provided by a larger group.

"Beware of any inexpensive health insurance," says Pollitz. "It will be too good to true. Health insurance is expensive."

Pollitz often tells a story about enrolling a fictitious, 46-year-old, breast cancer "survivor" of seven years, in order to test different health plans in Miami and Albany, N.Y. In Miami, out of seven plans tested, one company turned her down flat (illegal in Florida), one offered limited coverage and five offered policies ranging from about $300 to $1200 per month. In Albany, the same imaginary enrollee landed offers from all 10 health insurance plans but at much more affordable rates: $200 to $400. What HIPAA does for individual insurance buyers is guarantee renewability. In short, if you had an individual plan in place before the cancer diagnosis, it cannot be canceled.

Similarly, experts offer a helpful note in regard to small(er) businesses: Your co-workers, who might be good friends or family members, cannot lose their health insurance because you were sick. Geographically speaking, each state has its own department of insurance with toll-free telephone lines. Many states also run insurance-related Web sites that are worthy, if at times a bit klunky. You might try: http://fishercenter.georgetown.edu/genetic/discrimination/ for more help than you'll likely need.

Keeping Yourself Covered... and Current

Here's how to aim for—and receive—the best care and coverage from your health insurance provider.

- Keep exact records of all medical expenses. If you are too sick or fatigued, hire a health-claims processing firm if you can possibly afford it. It may pay for itself quickly, plus reduce greatly the load on a loved one.
- Send your claims in on time.
- If your claim is denied, appeal it. And appeal it. And appeal it again if you must. One college friend of mine, who's battled insurance companies for years, says working with insurance claims is like a stare-down, or what he calls "a wear-down." He who blinks first or gives up on claims first, loses.

Of special note for cancer patients: Don't settle for an insurance carrier denying use of "experimental" drugs or other treatments. State laws are becoming more progressive to allow consumers access to new treatment options that might be slow to pass federal approval.

For instance, some chemo drugs are officially approved for one type of cancer but routinely and effectively used by physicians to attack other tumors. As a result, insurance companies might try to deny the cost of those drugs for other uses. In this case it pays to inform the insurer that you plan to hire an attorney (one experienced in insurance matters). The National Coalition of Cancer Survivorship reports that "courts have generally sided with cancer patients in these circumstances."

Fighting: How (and When) to Fight Job Discrimination

Whether at your old job or a new one, if you do feel subject to discrimination because of your cancer diagnosis or treatment, there are several options to consider. The first step is to review the employer's usual policies for resolving such issues. An informal approach can often be the most effective.

If you need some flex time, seek the direct supervisor most able to gauge how it will affect a department or company's workload. Get that person on your side. If your employer offers accommodations, "don't take it lightly," says Barbara Hoffman of the NCCS. That offer might work in the employer's favor if the matter goes to court.

Keeping careful written records of any job actions is important, including such paperwork as past positive evaluations or being removed from the public interaction part of a position. There are deadlines to keep in mind for filing any formal complaint. The U.S. Equal Employment Opportunity Commission allows 180 days for filing, but if you work for the federal government you have only 45 days.

Still, experts say, most cancer survivors will do themselves a good turn by pausing before filing any formal complaint, including a lawsuit. Settling the matter out of court tends to lead to less animosity with your current employer—or questions from a future employer at a fraction (even zero) of the legal costs.

THAT WAS THEN, THIS IS NOW...

Back in 1996, Amgen, the California-based biotech firm, commissioned a survey of 500 (employed) cancer survivors, 100 supervisors and 100 co-workers of cancer survivors. The results provide a sobering perspective of on-the-job bias, just a decade ago: While researchers found that 81 percent of the survivors felt their jobs helped them maintain emotional stability during cancer diagnosis and treatment, the survey also showed supervisors were likely to overstate a survivor/worker's lost time and productivity. For instance: 85 percent of supervisors said fatigue was a major side effect suffered by cancer survivors on the job, while 58 percent of the survivors cited the problem. Some 75 percent of the supervisors said they thought the survivors experienced potentially life-threatening infection, fever or low white blood cell counts; but only 41 percent actually reported such side effects.

Donna Doneski, who works as a communications manager at the National Coalition for Cancer Survivorship in Silver Spring, Md., remembers a business magazine survey during the same time frame that revealed a surprisingly large number of respondents who still considered cancer to be contagious.

"I mean, 'No, you can't catch it,'" says Doneski. "People with cancer are more outspoken today on the subject of leading normal lives. That's progress, but getting health insurance or your job back still depends on who you are, where you are and what your job is."

The Money, Honey: Resources

National Coalition for Cancer Survivorship (NCCS)
(301) 650-9127; www.canceradvocacy.org
NCCS's promotes awareness of issues affecting cancer survivors. It is a superb clearinghouse with a savvy Web site and national experts on call.

Cancer Information Service
1-800-4-CANCER or 1-800-422-6237
A program of the National Cancer Institute (NCI). Nationwide telephone service for cancer patients and their families and friends. The staff answers questions (in English or Spanish) and sends free National Cancer Institute booklets about cancer. They also provide local resources and services.   www.cancer.gov

Job Accommodation Network
1-800-ADA-WORK or 1-800-232-9675
A free service of the President's Committee on Employment of People with Disabilities. It helps employers create accommodations for disabled employees.

www.healthinsuranceinfo.net/diabetes_and_health_insurance.pdf
Offers a wealth of modern guides and wisdom about getting, keeping and maximizing health insurance (though written for the diabetes community.) Offers a key guide for all to state insurance high risk pools.

Amercian Cancer Society
1-800-ACS-2345
Ask for the free booklet, "Your Job, Insurance and the Law."

RESOURCES continued...

Cancer Care, Inc.
1-800-813-HOPE or 1-800-813-4673
www.cancercare.org
Provides free help to cancer patients by offering information on cancer treatments, financial assistance, and other support services.

America's Health Insurance Plans (AHIP)
(202) 778.3200
www.hiaa.org/consumer
Its members include the large, sprawling health insurance companies and HMOs that people love to criticize, yet here they're giving back: The association and site provide insurance guides for survivors and consumers on topics such as health insurance costs, managed care, disability income, long-term care, and medical savings accounts.

U.S. Equal Employment Opportunity Commission (EEOC)
1-(800) 669-4000
Offers specific information about ADA (disability and illness) requirements affecting employees in the workplace.
Equal Employment Opportunity Commission
P.O. Box 7033
Lawrence, KS 66044
www.eeoc.gov/ada/adahandbook.html

CHAPTER 9

My Cancer Story (+3 years): The Sequel

RE-INTRO, RE-ENTRY

Two years since diagnosis, and I am cancer-free. Don't call myself a survivor...yet; feels too early. Don't call myself a "warrior," either. That's for the charity-fund appeal and pink-ribbon ad-campaign writers. But I've taken nine months of treatment ("We're gonna pound you," my radiation doc said); recovered from life-saving surgery with most of my body intact ("Don't stop cutting till you see the table," my colorectal surgeon said [in jest]); adopted a child; and I have started hugging my family and friends a bit harder.

Call me middle-aged guy in remission—make that recovery—because the way I see it, remission only means temporary absence of disease. Call me healthy but wary. Been bouncing back and forth from the U.S. to London, where [my wife] Paula is once again working as associate producer on the *Harry Potter* films. Been writing again, even some new kinds of stuff for a documentary I'm trying to get made. Been getting used to getting cancer behind me, even if it'll always seem ahead of me. Also been getting used to being a new dad, to giving all sorts of care at all hours to Baby Josh, kind of like Paula did for me. Still don't feel, though, that beating advanced colon cancer has made me "a better man." Even if I am, I've noticed, more apt to sign off letters, cards, and notes with "love."

PULP FRICTION

...Whirrrr-chop-chop-vrruuuuuuuhhhh!!! Got a juicer the other week, a bona fide institutional kind that weighs a ton, cost nearly $300, and grinds the goodness out of pretty much anything that grows on trees or out of the ground. *Vruhhhh-chop.* There's no scientific proof of freshly extracted juice adding 6.2 years to my life or anything; just advice from a good friend from Tulsa and a reasoned attempt to keep things that shouldn't be growing inside me from growing inside me.

RACE FOR MY CURE

SCENE: EXTERIOR: *Glinting, early-a.m., late-spring sun, Boulder, Colorado. Heli-cam ESTABLISHING SHOT, rolls east over the Foothills of the Rockies, panning over thousands of Lycra-clad runners (and walkers) and civilian-dressed road race officials milling about, near the intersection of 30th Street and Iris Ave., near the STARTING LINE of the 26th Annual Bolder Boulder 10K race.... Police barricades and scores of port-o-potties are lined up all along the staging areas leading to the pushoff point. PUSH shot of runner awkwardly trying to pin race number on to T-shirt with safety pins....*

EXTERIOR: *CLOSE-UP on AUTHOR, ME, 46-year-old colon cancer survivor, clad in bicycle shorts, T-shirt, sunglasses, new New Balance 860 running shoes... walking alone, slowly, toward start, one of 44,000 people who would enter the race this day. Tightening the Velcro straps on my warning/orange mesh jersey/vest—the one I'm wearing not for colon cancer awareness, but so my wife might find me during the run amid tens of thousands of non-survivors....*

CUT TO: *Rows of nervous runners moving slowly toward the starting line, like slaughterhouse cattle, only better dressed, and with lots less fat on their bones....*

CLOSE-UP: *MACRO on my right leg, and my right hand, grabbing the instep and top of my right foot. Bending back the foot—and knee—in a faux stretch that I'm doing mostly because everyone else is doing it. I'm a part-time runner, not a stud. I'm stretching to pass the time till the starter's gun goes off, not really to prevent the pain and fatigue I'll soon feel.*

Wondering, now, with fewer than five minutes till my "wave" starts the race, whether I've trained long-and-hard enough for a 6.2-mile run... at altitude. Knowing that I've spent six weeks or so training; but that I also don't expect to set any speed records this morning. My main goal: to finish. My second goal: to finish in less than an hour. (I'd clocked the race at 53 minutes back in 1999, pre-diagnosis.) Gun goes off. We start....

Lagging in the first mile, it seems, because I keep looking for the first water or Gatorade station stop.... Thirsty already; heavy legged. Gaining ground and speed in mile 3; especially after seeing Paula and Joshua, waiting patiently—and waving wildly—from in back of the Moe's Bagels shop, not 35 yards away.... I have my own cheeering section, I'm thinking, which translates to a short boost of energy to crest the hill on 13th Street....

Heading out of mile 5 and toward the home stretch on Folsom (toward the University of Colorado Buffaloes football stadium), and cursing the last hill that tries to Slow Us Down... realizing that I'm going to finish the race. Without stopping. Not a marathon, but enough. Six point two miles...in 63 minutes. Not learning until a few weeks later that my place in said race was 17, 601 out of 44,000 or so who entered. So I didn't finish a sub-60 10K, but I did run a "huge" race, in the top half of the field...in a time that was only 8 minutes slower than Frank Shorter, former Olympic marathon gold medalist. So what if he's in his 50s now? So what if he's a bit injured? I was still close to him (sort of). And maybe it doesn't much matter about the time. I trained, and finished, and learned. This ain't no Olympic trial. This is a colorectal cancer patient's attempt to take back his life, in one small way, three years after surgery. To blend in, literally, with the masses. And to run like I meant it, if only for today; if only for a short while....

SYNOPSIS: *Training for a 10K—running 8-10 miles a week, helps take one's mind off of "being a cancer patient." In my case, I became a runner again, if only for 63 minutes. In my case, the run helped me turn a corner on the disease aftermath, to help place it, frame it, more personally in my past. I could be, for an hour again, "one" with the masses, the (seemingly) healthy masses.*

CHEESEBURGER IN PARADISE

"You ever get ticked at me that you ate healthy all those years, and I didn't..." asks Geoff on a rare day of candor-studded best-friend banter, "and you got cancer?" Truth is, I don't get ticked at Geoff for that; I actually worry about his health. And he is allowed to say stuff like this, we agree, because his mom died of cancer when he was thirteen (and his dad, of diabetes complications, three years later). Have another bacon-cheese, Pal-o-mine.

CELEBRITY AND MY CANCER

Walking down skinny England's Lane, six weeks posttreatment, passing by a suitably Brit street sign: DEAD SLOW PLEASE—CHILDREN. Eyeing a guy wearing, of all things on a warm day, a red beret. Thinking I wouldn't bug the guy in New York or L. A., but this is London for chrissakes, and he isn't exactly blending in. I introduce myself to Tim Burton, without going googly or mentioning *Beetlejuice*, and end up inviting him to the premiere of *Harry Potter*. Then I speed-dial Paula to warn her what I've done without checking with any Warner Bros. honchos.

"You've lost your filter," she says. Meaning I'll say pretty much anything I want these days, to pretty much anybody. Even to a guy who had the gall to remake *Planet of the Apes* with Marky Frickin' Mark.

"HE'S LIVIN'"
[Excerpt from Paula's journal]

Back in England, I find I'm living with a forty-four-year-old teenager. Curt won't be where he doesn't want to be; or with who he doesn't want to be with. He's spontaneous and seizing the moment, not wasting time with small talk, pretending he's interested. He went to a play on a whim on Friday...*Rent* (again)...with some college kids he didn't know who had an extra cheap ticket to spare. He ran into them in Leicester Square. I tell him I was worried. Couldn't reach him for hours. "I'm livin'!" he said, and thank God he is.

WORDS YOU DON'T WANT TO HEAR

"...She will be cremated today after the medical specialists learn what they can to assist other warriors against cancer." – E-mail from a friend, about another friend, on a day I wasn't planning to think about my cancer. Much.

WORDS YOU WANT TO HEAR

"I recently read your articles this spring and was compelled to write to you to express how I was moved by your story and your writing. I will keep you in my prayers. If there is anything I can provide from my meager life in the Midwest, please don't hesitate to contact me. Very Truly Yours, Chris Jensen" Didn't contact him; he provided it anyway.

SOMEBODY ELSE'S TROUBLE

Every other Thursday, when I read the BBC.co.uk series by science writer Ivan Noble, about the malignant "tumour" that's found a home in his skull, I...read...every...word...incredibly...slowly. More slowly, perhaps,

179

than anything I've ever read on my crappy Apple laptop. As if by doing so, I'm showing this guy in his mid-thirties—newly married with a baby daughter for God's sake—some extra respect. Or by my doing so maybe his "fast-growing" tumor will somehow grow more slowly. Because, as he says, he doesn't expect it to go away anytime soon. Not to compare, but I heard the word "curable" from at least one doctor during my diagnosis.

Noble heard no such thing from his esteemed neurosurgeon. "There are no good brain tumours to have, [the neurosurgeon] said, but if there were, mine would not be one of them." [postscript: Noble died in early 2005.]

NEW LANG SYNE
12/27/02
TO: Chris and Monica
FROM: curtpmail@aol.com
----

dear monica and chris,

i went skating the other day, skated on the same rink i skated on two years ago this week, when i found out i had cancer....

i went skating the other day, skated with the same friend i skated with two years ago in boulder, the one i didn't have the strength to tell that awful day i just found out i had colon cancer....

i went skating the other day; did laps around the rink one way, then the other, while watching a mom with her 2-year-old and his double runners—double runners that didn't seem to be working very well.

i went skating the other day, as a new dad with clean CT scans....

i went skating the other day, thinking about Joshua joining me next year on that rink in Colorado; thinking about Paula who will be there worrying if he's going too fast around the corners, and I'll be thinking, "all's pretty much right with the world," thanks to good doctors, truly great friends like you, and some powerful, prayerful, medicine.

i went skating the other day, and this time the Christmas tunes didn't sound tinny, false, taped: this time they echoed off the ice and into my ears, into my heart.

now, everybody off the damn ice, so they can scrape it...clean it...and let everybody start over...doncha' know?

happy new year, guys, to you and your amazing family,

love, curt

THREE TIMES A YEAR
[Excerpt From P.'s journal]

I'm in a lot better place now, I guess because it's January. Next scans aren't till the end of April. That's because Dr. [Allen] Cohn says, "every three to four months (for the first two years after surgery, then every six)." And Curt's figured out, if we stretch it out till four, that's one less per year, plus less radiation.

I find myself now living my life with this benchmark. So far relieved, and filled with joy, but as the weeks pass, feeling the dread that so slowly creeps up on me, as the next trip home gets closer. When we sit in the oncologist's office, trying to anticipate and read into his every expression...hearts-are-racing...then learning he hasn't read them yet; will be right back....Trying to hear the pace of his footsteps as he returns to see if they will give me any insight as to the news about to be delivered. Do we get to continue our lives as they are—so full of love and joy, and our new baby, Joshua...or do we put on our gear again and go into the fire and fight for life?

AS A JAYBIRD

One thing I've noticed: Ever since cancer, ever since surgery, ever since I've owned a post-op stoma protruding ever so slightly from my torso, I don't flit about the house so often as I used to, naked.

MY ADOPTION STORY

You don't enter the world of adoption lightly. But in the summer of '96, after Paula almost died following an ectopic pregnancy that exploded, sort of, into her uterine insides, where some nasty arteries reside and where she internally bled quarts of blood for way too long before they figured out why her blood pressure had dropped to "0" ...we thought of it.

No, you don't enter the world of adoption lightly, so we have been in it heavily now, for two years running. And we have a son who wasn't born when I had my Big Run with colorectal cancer, and what am I going to tell him about it, not yet sure. Yet when he sees me in the shower wearing a Band Aid-colored bag on my lower torso, he's gonna ask eventually, so I will tell him what makes sense, what is true, along with the fact that were it not for my cancer, or Paula's ectopic, we may not have found Joshua Daniel, ever.

FALSE ALARM?

Waking on a cold morning, early winter, with a twinge astride my right testicle that ranges from groin to lower torso...uh-oh. Feels a little like a groin pull, but higher, and connected to the dull, lingering pains I feel in my lower abdomen when I do push-ups or other ab work (not that I do a lot of "ab work"). Surgery scar tissue, maybe, or worse? Make a note to ask about this pain at the next CT-scan checkup in two months.

THE FIRE THIS TIME

"You smell something burning?" Paula says [July '02]. "You see the fire out there?" Hard to believe, hard to miss, but after three years of trying to get pregnant, and two years of trying to adopt, we finally bring our seven-month-old baby home from his poverty-ravaged Guatemala...and the neighborhood's nearly on fire.

Fewer than five hours after landing, on Josh's first night in the U.S., without warning, a Colorado wildfire erupts and crawls down the nearby foothills toward Wonderland Lake—and our backyard. "Unfrickin' believable," I'm thinking from the upstairs back bedroom window, "it's not burning itself out..." Instead, it's looking like molten lava moving over drought-starved grasses. Phone rings, we pick up. Friends up the road, forced out of their home. They're on the way over. Paula's in bed with Joshua, trying to let him sleep....

Phone rings again later; I pick up. "You are being advised to evacuate...." recorded message from the sheriff's office drones. It's 2:00 am. and we're haphazardly packing photos and bags furiously...aided by Nancy, Cory, Amelia, and Aidan and their Lab/Rhodesian Ridgeback puppy that doesn't have a clue. No time to ponder the tragicomic timing—"Do we take the [big] wedding photo or the album??"—as the next chapter of our storybook life unfolds. We stay put. I stay up until 4:30 a.m. Next day we learn four hundred acres got torched; nobody got killed; our property got a free pass....Welcome home, Son.

THE SCANS GAME

Driving south on Highway 36, heading out of the Boulder foothills and down to Denver to see my oncologist, my reader of CT scans of abdomen, of pelvis, of chest, who checks for signs of rogue cells. Passed the one-year mark okay, then the year and a half...but for some reason the year and nine months has me jittery. Maybe it's because I'm a father now, maybe it's because I had that twinge...(though ex-cancer patients, I learn, are forever mistaking twinges for recurrence).

Here we go...and turns out I have no reason to worry. No "evidence for...metastatic disease"; no changes, apparently, from the study four months prior. Dr. Cohn walks into the exam room and starts chatting with me about my recent stint in England. "You likin' it over there?" Good news. If I had cancer signs, he wouldn't be talking tourism. "You're healthy," he says. I ask him to repeat this into my Sony microcassette that I have placed on the chair next to me ...(in case of bad news and my note-taking/thinking/reasoning all going to hell). "He's healthy!" Dr. Cohn says loudly to the Sony and thus to Paula, who will hear this tape at home after the baby wakes up. I smile as if I knew all along all would be okay (as if) and hop out to the car to call home. (You don't shout the good news into a cell phone in the Rocky Mountain Cancer Center.... Too many ill patients in attendance.)

Now I'm back on the road, rolling north, toward Highway 36 and home, feeling like I have just graduated from something big, singing along to a Springsteen CD, pounding the steering wheel as a snare drum, or cymbal, as if I'm aping Tony Soprano.

> *"These are better days, bay-buh /*
> *These are better days it's true /*
> *These are better days, bay-buh /*
> *There's better days shining through."*

SEX AND MY CANCER

Viagra this, Viagra that. Didn't think, when I was fighting cancer so fiercely, that it would have made a huge deal if I had come out of surgery okay but learned I'd be Viagra-dependent for life. I was flat-out wrong (and glad I had crack surgeons). Spontaneous sex is thrilling, more so when you realize you nearly lost the chance to have it. Even so, to come clean, I don't have it nearly as often as I used to: The twice-a-week standard I've seen quoted so often hasn't applied to me or my partner, if she doesn't mind me saying so, for at least six months. And it doesn't totally have to do with us being new parents, zonk-tired, up at 4:00 a.m. It's partly due to the lack of spontaneity I feel when it comes to sex, now that I have one more thing (a fairly big thing, actually) to consider...besides time, place, baby feeding, who's gotta get up in the morning. I mean, I gotta think about going into the john, emptying, folding, and medi-taping my ostomy bag to my belly so it doesn't get in the way of, sorry, there's no other way to say it, Hon, thrusting.

GOLF AND MY CANCER

Standing on the first tee at St. Andrews Old Course, 6:30 a.m., under leaden Scottish skies, one year after surgery, alone with my friend Renny on a course not yet open, here because he's pulled some strings, told some sad-true tale of an American friend who battled bowel cancer and came out of it alive, who's now waggling his Big Berthas and itching to play a round by the Firth of Forth (at the first available opportunity). As if the links gods are watching, kid you not a whit, there's a break in the clouds and the sun decides to join us on golf's shrine, if only for a moment.

THE ENDORSEMENT: THE BAG

Friend asks how everything's going—I can tell he means with the stoma, the ileostomy, the not-exactly-colostomy I had during surgery.... "Okay," I say. "I go to the gym, bike, hike, eat pretty much anything...." Turns out his mom's friend has a bag, got blocked up and she had to go to the hospital, twice, from peanuts. Twice??!! I'd give up the peanuts if I got blocked up once. Don't wanna know how the thing gets flushed.

CHOOSING MY RELIGION

A Jewish family friend writes: "I don't know if you remember me, but I do you—When my mom had breast cancer, I didn't understand a lot of what she was going through. Reading your articles allowed me to feel it for the first time.... God chooses people he knows can handle it. He chose you...."

Thanks, God. Got my colon carved out in an eight-hour surgery, lost forty-five pounds and nine months of my life in a freakish/mawkish/radiated/toxic-chemical/narcotics-infused blur of an assault, and as far as I know, Osama's still doing fine, humpin' it round the Afghan/Pakistani border, with a leaky frickin' kidney. Still I pray.

NAP TIME

Sometimes when Joshua sleeps in my arms, his warm head cradled in the crook of my elbow, I want to cry for the joy I feel.

Or maybe for the pain I didn't let myself feel when I thought I might die ahead of my time. And his.

STATS ALL, FOLKS

Two years post-op, two and a half since diagnosis, sitting on Doc Cohn's tissue-paper-covered leather table one more time. Learning, on April 22, 2003, that there are no lesions visible in my latest set of scans. He says I am healthy, then serves up a best-supporting statistic: "Eighty percent of the people who develop a recurrence [of colorectal cancer] get it in the first two years," he says. Which means just 20 percent develop it later.

Handshakes and hugs all around; pretty good odds, I figure. Until later that day, when I realize: Before I was first diagnosed, people like me, ex-colitis patients, had less than a 20 percent chance of developing colon cancer in the first dang place…. At the three-year mark [and at the big five-year CT in '06], my scans again appear medically "unremarkable." Which I—on the other hand, a few years after dealing with an elusive, shadowy death rattle—find rather remarkable.

Quick call to family, with Paula at my side; then dial best pal Geoff in L. A.

"I don't have can-cerrrrr, I don't have can-cerrrrr," I sort of white-man-rap at him. "I don't have can-cerrrrrrr!" Pause. Then he answers: "This month."

Letters to the...Author

Date: Fri, 4 Jun 2004 07:50:15 EDT
From: <Scou@aol.com>
To: <curtpmail@aol.com>
Subject: another article

"Cancer Deaths Down in U.S., Report Finds"

WASHINGTON (June 3) - More Americans are surviving cancer for five years or more and cancer rates overall are steadily declining, according to the latest annual report on cancer in the United States issued on Thursday.

Talk About It
*   Post Messages
*   Top News Boards

[Author's note: Yes, Scou@aol.com. We will, Scou. We will Talk About It.]

From the time I learned I had advanced colorectal cancer, through nine months of treatment, through writing about what it felt like, through the 3-year mark of "all-clear" follow-up tests and scans, I received more emotional letters, emails and postcards, by far, than I did in 43 years of life prior to my life-threatening diagnosis. Writing, it turns out, can be more than therapeutic for many a cancer patient. It can be life-affirming. A handful of the most memorable, and of those perhaps most helpful to other survivors, appears below*.

From *Esquire* magazine's July , 2001 issue, letters-to-the-editor page:

"Fighting Cancer"

Our May issue...featured the first part of an ongoing series by Curtis Pesmen on his battle with colon cancer ("My Cancer Story: Part One").

I picked up Esquire several times this past week, and each time I put it down. Fear made me do it—the fear that the word cancer spreads. But finally Pesmen's words seduced me, and I found myself devouring his piece, wanting to understand every emotion and physical sensation he felt. Part of that was self-defense; part of it came from reading a piece that pierced the armor I carry to shield myself from the idea of disease. When I finished, I picked up the phone and called my doctor, whom I had-n't seen in a couple of years, and said, "I'm thirty-five, and I want a full checkup." He said, "Wise move." I said a friend suggested it. If courage and bravery count for anything, Pesmen will kick cancer's ass.

—Richard Abate, New York, NY

(Note: some names have been abbreviated or deleted, for privacy reasons.)

Letter from a stranger, April, 2001:

Dear Mr. Pesmen,

It's Easter Sunday morning as I write.... Although I'm not a religious person, my faith in humankind is a bit restored as a result of your writing Part I in Esquire. Like your friend's daughter wished you, ..."I hope you fight off your cancer."

On an action-taking note, I'm 62 years of age and tomorrow I will call for a sigmoidoscopy exam. So thanks for being the impetus for my doing what is overdue. With sincere wishes for a full recovery and the very best for you and your wife.

--T.R.

Letter from a friend, April, 2001, one week after stressful, successful, eight-hour surgery:

Dear Curt and Paula,

Well, I'm sure you have heard every bit of consolation, hope and now finally praise. Count me among the grateful. Thousands thanking God this day and just about every after for the good news that broke last week.

There are few people in the world who bring with them such calm and good will as Curt brings with him. I don't know if that is because we have sat next to each other at various functions and he lets me yammer on, that could be. But I have heard other people say the same thing about him and I am inclined to believe it is a genuine good disposition. Count me among the fortunate for knowing a wonderful person like Curt.

For two people to be in such an extreme position and display their love to each other in caring and patience, and for showing the immortal strength of love, count me among the believers.

Before you guys left [before the diagnosis], Paula and I were talking about her particular skill in the work place...and her ability to keep a cool head and manage multiple tethers, numbers, personalities and information. For Paula's being able to handle the circus of appoint-ments, treatments and doctors without flinching or buckling, count me among the amazed.

While you may find this a bit much, I didn't know how else to let you both know how much you mean to me and just how happy I am that Curt is on the mend. I realize that there is more work ahead for you both, but know that we are still thinking about you, and will continue to root for speed on your road to recovery.

Love you both, and so very happy—

Booey

From an old colleague, young cancer survivor, and friend, May, 2001:

Dear Curt,

That's a hell of a way to have a two-part [sic] feature in Esquire!

Curt, I am so sorry to hear about your cancer. I read your pieces with my heart in my mouth and tears in my eyes. So much of what you said mir-rored my own experience with breast cancer four years ago. And, although the whole thing completely sucks, I'm so grateful that you have a strong, loving partner with whom to go through it.

One thing you didn't mention was whether you had friends or support group pals who also had cancer and are our age. I felt with breast cancer that, because it's so politicized and so feminist-y, I fell into this ready made community of supportive women and it really helped me. Just to have someone to talk to, to vent with, someone who is not your spouse and doesn't have quite that emotional investment, someone who is going through it or has gone through it, someone who can hear your darkest fears without panicking.

And I wanted you to know that if you ever need to talk to someone about [being] a young person with cancer, my number is at the top of this page. That's it. I wish you the best of luck, the best of health, the best of love and all the strength you need.

Much love,

Peggy O., California

From a not-quite-friend of a friend, May, 2001:

Dear Curt,

You may not know me...but my father was diagnosed with a rare form of skin cancer when he was just approaching 45 and I was 17 at the time and I can remember that it was the 1st time I saw my father cry. Sometimes my Mom and Dad would just sit on the couch and start crying together. I could not really understand that at the time and it made me feel so awkward to see that and not know what to say or do. I remember the frustration in their voices...and it seems like everybody is polite to you but also scared to talk to you in fear that you may want to talk about "it," and that would just make us so uncomfortable.

Mmmhhh, let's think on that one... makes "us" uncomfortable?? Hell, there is nothing wrong with "us" now, is there? What about the person with the darn cancer, ever thought how uncomfortable they are—physically, emotionally and overall just uncomfortable knowing this damn cancer has invaded their body without their consent and often for a long time without them ever knowing?

Have we ever stopped to think how uncomfortable "YOU" must be? No, we tend to be selfish and think of us first and foremost and yes, then there is the thought of others...and how sorry we may feel about them and how tragic that someone we know may be sick, but followed right away by the afterthought, "Thank God it is not me!" How selfish can we get? It wasn't until a couple years ago that I understood that concept of thinking when I witnessed a good friend of mine die of AIDS. Not a pretty sight....

Curt—you and Paula are in my deepest prayer tonight and every night and I sure hope that I will have the pleasure of getting to meet both of you one day.

Best wishes,

S.E., North Carolina

From a friend of a friend, who lives in St. Louis

Dear Curt,

When I had cancer five years ago, I was sure I'd be dead by now. I spent a lot of hours crying about my children being raised without me, etc., and giving my sister and my husband lots of instructions. I even listed the single friends who would make acceptable stepmothers. Any time anyone told me I looked good—a complete lie as my skin was green during chemo, and my hair is one of my best features—I would say, "Open Casket."

Ignore everyone's advice, but here's some anyway: Avoid all books that tell you to have a positive attitude. Wallow—you've more than earned it. Wishing you all the best. If I had crystals, I'd use them—that is, after someone explained to me what the hell they're supposed to do.

Part of my nightmare was that my kids were 8 and 5, and one of my parents died when I was 8, but if we're going to throw around cancer psycho-babble, my guess is that losing a body part, like a breast, is a pretty tangible daily reminder. Even to someone who has had her plastic surgery redone numerous times.

Not that I'm trying to one-up you or anything. Here's an anecdote to cheer you up: The goofball husband of an old friend of mine had testic-ular cancer the same time I had breast cancer. Whenever he felt espe-cially freaked out, he would call me to "commisserate," but really to work into the conversation that his cancer had a 98 percent cure rate, unlike mine. Not that I'm the sort of person to hold a grudge.

Best, Jill F.

From *Esquire*'s September, 2001, issue, letters page:
"The Continuing Battle"

July also brought the third installment in Curtis Pesmen's ongoing account of his fight with colorectal cancer ("My Cancer Story").

I am forty. I have brain cancer. I was diagnosed in April and was operated on five days later, and have seven radiation treatments to go. Hats off to Pesmen for sharing his experience with us all. It isn't easy to read, but cancer isn't easy to have. I've learned a lot, but mostly that fatigue and nausea are the two most misrepresented words in the English language. Good stuff, but damn, I'm mad. Seven months ago, I ran a marathon. And I guess, just like Pesmen, I don't want to die.

—T.T., Richmond, Va.

From a writer friend in New York, with whom I had some tough words in the spring of 2001:

Dear Curt,

Thanks a million for calling last night.... You asked me why I wanted to reach out to you when I haven't done so with others in the past. I think the simple answer is: It's about you. With other people I've often been afraid that my expressions of sympathy would sound like I was just projecting my own fears, like the way people who cry at weddings are overwhelmed by their own romantic ideals, not the reality of someone else's life. I've been afraid there was something phony about forging a close relationship with someone only after they contracted a serious disease. Even in your case I couldn't help wondering if you thought your writer friends might try to use you in a Mitch Albom-esque way.

The difference here is that I know you. We may be closer to other people than we are to each other, but I feel for sure that over the years we've moved past the friends-of-friends status to being just friends, and I certainly know you well enough to have genuine feelings for you as a person.... And it's not just a personal loss for me; I know too how many people you've touched and what the loss of you would mean to them.

So now back to our mutual insensitivities: what have we learned from all this? How about: I promise not to say any more obnoxious things if you promise not to have any more cancer.

Still your friend,
Ben

From a distant cousin of mine, to whom I now feel closer, spring, 2001:

I bought Esquire to read Curt's article, and I did not even wait to get home to read it. Just sat in my car and wept. It is brilliant – searingly honest, the story of a man who just does not have time to tell anything but the truth. I hope it will be some comfort to him to know that he is bringing comfort to others, those who are ill and those who will someday be ill (and that's everyone) with his story.
–Nell

From a distant friend of mine, to whom I now feel closer, spring, 2001:

What can I say about the article but WOW! I know it left me exhausted and speechless just reading it.... I can't possibly imagine living through it!! The one thing that I keep thinking about is how wonderful it is that Curt is able to tell his story. Throughout our ordeal 8 years ago with our daughter Barbara, we had so very many well-wishers but in reality no one truly wanted to hear the down and dirty details of what we were living through from birth to funeral. And I think it would have done me a lot of good to have been able to vent and tell in detail what was happening. But in truth even my very best friends probably didn't feel as if they could handle such details coming from me and so John and I and the family were left storing them away and keeping them to ourselves. The writing of this series for Curt, as extremely difficult as it must have been, was most probably also a cleansing (I hope) for him also.

All my love to you both,
Erin

An email from a friend in New York, upon learning of the death of a young friend of mine, July, 2004:

Curt,

You know, I'm beginning to believe that it's the norm and not heroic for people to keep fighting and stay optimistic when they are really ill (not that I can tell YOU how people act when they are ill...). But truly, I've yet to run in to anyone who has a dire illness who DOES-N'T rally to live and fight on. Part of this is because we don't see them when they are curled up in a ball in the corner of the room petrified of what's to come.

But I do find this so inspiring.... Imagine: it's not "normal" for a person who is dying to become morbid; it is "normal" for the human spirit to fight back and stay "up" for everyone around them. Remember the last thing you wanted was for people to think of you as "Cancer Boy," so the only way to insure that is to act like you are NOT sick.... Makes sense, no?

Anyway, she did fight the fight and what is amazing to me is that she continued to accomplish writing a book.... I can't even get myself to paint my apartment.

Are you okay?
--H.

From an old pal, ex-girlfriend, and breast cancer survivor, who read an article of mine and reached out my way, spring 2007:

Curt-

I always felt badly about the fact that you were the unfortunate recipient of so much of my own unfiltered deeply-depressing stuff I couldn't talk to my other "real-world" friends about...that they didn't want to hear and/or didn't understand. [You know,] its sadly too rare that we ever get to know what "exes" really thought about anything.

xo, S.

From my father, 72, after an early-morning airport departure following his four-day visit during my chemo.

Dearest Children,

You two have given me such optimism-courage-support I feel like I'm the one who is winning the battle!

I love you both so much—

Dad

From *Esquire* magazine's October, 2001 issue, letters page:
"On the Road to Recovery"

> *In August, Pesmen continued with the fourth part of his series on his fight against colon cancer.*

I have been an *Esquire* subscriber for more than thirty years. I keep renewing because I feel that Esquire deals intelligently with issues affecting men. My faith has been reinforced by your publication of Curtis Pesmen's "My Cancer Story." I was diagnosed with colon cancer more than seven years ago. I have read all of Pesmen's articles and think that he has been able to convey the emotions that I felt during my diagnosis and treatment. His article, however, is just the beginning of the fight, as cancer is never cured but only goes into remission.

For the rest of his life, every little ache, fever or other change in his body will bring concerns that the monster has returned. If it does, as has mine has, a new set of feelings will come. I realize that I will eventually die of cancer and it is important to make every day enjoyable. It appears that Pesmen has the most important tool needed to cope with his illness and prolong his life—a loving, caring, and supportive wife.

—T.B., Metairie, La.

Sources & Resources

The following survivor resources are meant to provide thoughtful or medically-based means to increase your chances of living longer, stronger. Some are well-known to doctors, nurses and patients; others are less-publicized but invaluable to caregivers and to those who've faced a tough diagnosis and didn't know quite where to turn. And still others offer little more than laughter. Necessary, helpful laughter.

A WORD ABOUT WEBSITES

While it's tough to obtain complete, unbiased cancer information from any one internet site, it is the rare patient who consults only one website. "A few good sites," is the educated survivors' goal. Too many may be daunting; too few not helpful enough. Used to be, cancer survivors and caregivers were cautioned that the best sites were those that were "neutral," and free of advertising. These days, though, it is generally recognized that information-rich websites incur legitimate costs in order to create and maintain current, helpful content. So even the "good guys" may need to run some ads for revenue alongside their listings, images or online articles. All links herein were functional as of late 2008.

GENERAL, PATIENT-FRIENDLY SOURCES

- The Colon Cancer Alliance (CCA)
  http://www.ccalliance.org calls itself a national advocacy group that represents "the voice of colorectal cancer survivors." It is also the patient-support partner of the National Colorectal Cancer Research Alliance (NCCRA), which was founded by NBC TODAY show co-anchor Katie Couric, cancer activist Lilly Tartikoff, and

the Entertainment Industry Foundation. For NCCRA patient trials info:
http://www.eifoundation.org/national/nccra/splash/index.html
For CCA: 877-422-2030 toll free

- The Colorectal Cancer Coalition (C3)
  http://www.fightcolorectalcancer.org is one of the few patient-oriented
  organizations devoted specifically to colorectal cancer, offering support, information and advocacy. It has a targeted area for research:
  with links to current clinical trials, plus helpful, plain-language inter-
  pretation of science-laden advances. A one-stop shop.

- The National Institutes of Health,
  http://www.nih.gov, is the government's main medical agency under
  the U.S. Department of Health and Human Services. Tax dollars bring
  us these very well designed, easy-to-navigate websites. The Health
  Information page, http://health.nih.gov/ and Medline Plus,
  http://www.nlm.nih.gov/medlineplus/ are logical, clear sites offering
  dozens of pages on clinical trial results, drug information, and medi-
  definitions. The latter is updated and is bilingual. Use the "search"
  box, *vominos*, to focus on your specific questions, or you may get dis-
  tracted by everything from eczema to rabies.

- A related site from the National Center for Complementary and
  Alternative Medicine (CAM), http://nccam.nih.gov/ keeps abreast of
  CAM by exploring current herbal and other practices, like acupuncture, in the context of rigorous science. Not limited to cancer treatments, but is helpful in detailing how complementary and alternative
  medicine researchers are trained; also, how some overlooked natural
  medicines are used (legally) in foreign countries.

- National Cancer Institute
  http://www.nci.nih.gov/ is another key federal agency, charged with
  "eliminating the suffering and death due to cancer." Its PDQ

(Physician Data Query) is NCI's comprehensive cancer database that contains thousands of peer-reviewed summaries of key research findings. Search for trials, follow results—a kind of cancer studies' box score. Alternate address for NCI information:
http://www.cancer.gov/

- Lance Armstrong Livestrong Foundation
http://www.livestrong.org The premise is simple, but with a few twists. Beyond the iconic yellow bracelets, the Armstrong community uses the profound celebrity power of a world-class athlete and Tour de France champ cancer survivor to fund an ever-growing team of cancer survivors and other supporters. With emphasis nearly always on survivorship, the programs and one-on-one sessions tackle issues related to cancer drugs, other meds, partner counseling, financial and insurance pressures, while helping patients find and enroll in clinical trials.

- American Cancer Society
www.cancer.org. For the colon cancer survivor, there are the personalized NexProfiler Treatment Options and Treatment Outcome tools, https://www.cancer.nexcura.com/Secure/ToolBox.asp?CB=267.
Fill out the questionnaire about your personal situation (it's free) and targeted information from scientific medical studies is offered. While not comprehensive, it is certainly a valuable tool for collating much of the latest research. Also valuable, same site, is the Medical Records Assistant. Printable forms help organize medical history, ask the right questions, and letters requesting info or authorizing the release of info. A sort-of free medi-secretary.

- CancerCare
http://www.cancercare.org/
"No one should have to face cancer alone," says this national non-profit group, which offers free wide-ranging advice. The range of serv-

ices is dizzying, but not limited to colorectal cancer issues. Support and guidance in English or Spanish are provided by social workers and online chat groups. Plus, this .org runs regular telephone workshops, which present specific solutions—for a variety of cancer patients' problems.

- United Ostomy Association
www.uaoo.org offers support, education, information and advocacy for those with intestinal or urinary stomas, pouches or "diversions." A great place to ask questions (anonymously, if desired), and also to keep up with the latest products serving the intestinally diverted.

- The American Gastroenterological Association offers a GI (gastro) doc locator, organized by state.
http://www.gastro.org/generalPublic.html

HELP VS. HYPE

When someone starts trying to sell you a "wonderful new" or "radical cure," head first to Quackwatch, an advocate site.
http://www.quackwatch.org/index.html

- The University of Texas, M.D. Anderson's Complementary/Integrative Medicine site, http://www.mdanderson.org/departments/cimer/ follows the ever-changing CAM frontier. Updated often, it offers relevant features like Drug Interaction and FDA Advisories.

- Memorial Sloan-Kettering's database,
http://www.mskcc.org/mskcc/html/11570.cfm. Offers exhaustive information on herbs, botanicals and other products. From one of the top cancer hospitals in the world http:/www.msk.org

SCIENCE-SKEWED SOURCES

- ACOR, www.acor.org, Association of Cancer Online Resources: Technical, at times tough to navigate, but offers quite helpful information about drugs and treatment protocols.

- PubMed, a service of the National Library of Medicine, includes over 15 million citations for biomedical articles back to the 1950's. www.ncbi.nlm.nih/pubmed

- http://www.nature.com/cancer/
  Nature Cancer Update is a bio-science heavy resource for cancer news, reviews and research from the Nature Publishing Group. Features include research, trial watch and research updates.

RESOURCES IN PRINT

10 BOOKS WORTH CUTTING DOWN TREES FOR...:

1] *What Your Doctor May Not Tell You About Colon Cancer*—Mark Pochapin, M.D., with a foreword by Katie Couric (Warner Books)

2] *Cancer Free: The Comprehensive Prevention Program, Prevent Cancer Guide*—by Sloan-Kettering doctors, Sidney Winawer, M.D., and Moshe Shike, M.D (Simon & Schuster)

3] *My Breast*—Joyce Wadler (Addison Wesley)

4] *It's Not About the Bike*—by Lance Armstrong with Sally Jenkins (Broadway Books). (A bettter read than *Every Second Counts*, his follow-up book)

5] *Healing Lessons*—Sidney J. Winawer, M.D., with Nick Taylor. (Little Brown) An unforgettable story of what transpires when one of the world's most renown digestive disease specialists, who works at Memorial Sloan-Kettering hospital in New York, finds out his wife – the love of his life – develops life-threatening stomach cancer and wishes to try alternative medical therapies.

6] *The Journey Through Cancer*—by Jeremy Geffen, M.D. (Crown Books) Helps readers through some of the toughest questions of survivorhood, like: How (and when) can I give my caregiver(s) a break? Does energy healing actually work? And, How do I want to be remembered in life?

7] *Cancer: Fight it With the Blood Type Diet*—by Peter J. D'Adamo (Putnam) Intriguing, if no longer as controversial as it was in the '90s. This book looks at how different diets help fight cancer, according to one's specific blood type. The author is a widely-known naturopath (doctor who mainly uses food and nutrients to heal) who, among other things, proposes "super-beneficials", which are foods for cancer-fighting-immunity boosts.

8] *Enter Sandman*—by Stephanie Williams (McWitty Press). Unlikely choice to make this list, because it's a novel. Also because the protagonist is a young woman who develops breast, not colon, cancer. Contains some of the best, evocative writing I've seen about how one's self image changes, over time, as chemotherapy and surgery take their toll on one's body…in this case, the body of a young, attractive, engaging and successful New York City woman—who happens to be a woman in love. Sadly, the author died of breast cancer, at age 33, in 2004.

9] *Man to Man*—by Michael Korda (Vintage). A no-nonsense, prostate cancer guide, conversational and brutally honest. He even criticizes the surgeon who "saved" him. That's refreshing. And medically respectable.

10] *Be Prepared: The Complete Financial, Legal, and Practical Guide for Living with a Life-Challenging Condition*—by David S. Landay (St. Martin's Press).

MAGAZINES

- *CURE: Cancer Updates, Research & Education*
  http://www.curetoday.com/ is a quarterly magazine that combines the science of cancer with warmth of observant patients writing about their experiences.

- *Coping Magazine*
  www.copingmag.com Besides providing day-to-day practical advice, *Coping* magazine is an official sponsor of National Cancer Survivors Day.

- *Natural Health*
  www.naturalhealthmag.com This reader-friendly magazine publishes practical and well-researched articles and opinions about some of the best natural medicine options around.

- *Natural Solutions*
  http://www.naturalsolutionsmag.com/index.cfm Although the title seems general enough, the magazine has, over the years, retained a keen anti-cancer sensibility in its articles and supplement reviews.

OTHER MEDIA

FILMS / MOVIES/ VIDEO

- Anything by The Marx Brothers

- *Healing and the Mind*, (1992) The six-part, PBS documentary, aired originally on public television and narrated by Bill Moyers, is a powerful look at overlooked powerful medicine, including the much wider use of acupuncture in our collective future.

- *The Doctor* (1991), stars William Hurt, offers patients a doctor's-eye view of what it feels like to make a shocking transition from tough doc to frightened patient...and to realize how much room there is for improvement in the everyday practices of doctors as well as in the halls of the very best hospitals, themselves.

- National Lampoon's *Animal House* (1979), starring John Belushi, Peter Riegert and Karen Allen, almost inarguably, launched a genre of over-the-top, at-times gross-out comedies that deliver, beside potentially immune-boosting biochemical changes, true belly laughter.

- *Old School* (2003), starring Will Ferrell, Luke Wilson and Vince Vaughan. You could say it's Animal House meets American Pie; I'll merely say it's a future classic in post-millennial comedic "film."

CD

- The EIF (Entertainment Industry Foundation), the Hollywood powerhouse fundraising and awareness group that funds the National Colorectal Cancer Research Alliance, has produced free patient-friendly CDs. Go to http://www.eifoundation.org/national/nccra/publiced/materials.asp for a free copy of Katie Couric's educational CD entitled "What you need to know." The name says it all. Included are dozens of .pdf files with authorative studies, charts, all levels of information specific to colon cancer. Mpg files show filmed commercials by celebs urging people to "get tested, this one can be cured." And of course, there is the famed celebrity-colonoscopy that Ms. Couric intimately and nobly shared with the world, at: kcolon.mpg.

EXTRA HELP

- The Air Care Alliance,
  http://www.aircareall.org/ for air transport that insurance doesn't cover. You might also get a lift on Corporate Angel Network, http://www.corpangelnetwork.org/patient/index.html, if you have an appointment at a recognized cancer treatment facility. The service needs three weeks notice but can't guarantee a seat. You can't bring life support equipment on the big plush seats either, but it's hitch-hiking high style.

- Needy Meds
  http://www.needymeds.org is a sort of Yellow Pages/ Yellow Book for information on free meds for those who qualify. Search the drug's Brand, Generic Name, the Manufacturer or the Program to find out criteria. Lack or lapse of insurance coverage usually qualifies a few months worth of costly tablets. Required paperwork and detailed instructions are also listed. Hey, it's free.

- CancerCare
  http://www.cancercare.org/pdf/ru/Bill_of_Rights.pdf helps inform patients and survivors of our rights.

Acknowledgements

Before this book could be written, a number of people had to set about saving my life in order that it might be written. With that in mind, my deepest, heartfelt gratitude goes to Daphne Haas-Kogan, M.D., Mark Lane Welton, M.D., Alan Venook, M.D., and Peter R. Carroll, M.D. I also give everlasting thanks to the nurses and support staffs (and to Pat Hunter) at the University of California-San Francisco Medical Center, and to Allen Cohn, M.D., and staff at Rocky Mountain Cancer Centers, Denver.

I am indebted, more than they know, to the Columbus and Williams clans in San Francisco, and to my amazing family closer to home. My parents, Harold and Sandra Pesmen, gave me the greatest gifts—life and love and a sense of self—but also gave me a sister, Beth, whose family has always been a pillar to me, and for me. I am grateful to all the friends and colleagues who offered their thoughts and prayers—and made more out-of-town visits than any patient or pal could imagine—in my harrowing year of treatment. Along with family members Jeanne Ward and B.J. Marsh, Laura and Phil Scott, Jeannie Austin and Curtis Carillo, our "family members" at 1492 Pictures and Warner Bros. in London and Los Angeles all provided inspiring light during a dark, dark year.

Among the many health care professionals who pitched in to help me spread my message, the staffs at the Jay Monahan Center for Gastrointestinal Health at New York Presbyterian Hospital/Weill Cornell Medical Center and Memorial Sloan-Kettering Cancer Center in Manhattan were as gracious as they were knowledgeable. Similarly, my dealings with Kevin Lewis at the Colon Cancer Alliance, and Priscilla Savary and Louise Bates at Colorectal Cancer Network, were both incisive and helpful. In the world of specialized medicine, the American Society of Colon and Rectal Surgeons graciously allowed me full access to pre-booked sessions—and the sometimes startling images associated with them—at the 2004 annual meeting in Dallas.

Heartfelt thanks also go to dear friends Geoff Hansen and Barb Brabec, Todd Neal and Gretchen Hoag, the Devereuxs, Mitch Engel, Pete and Toby Christensen, Ed McNally and Monique Martin, Rose and Tim Healion, Jerry and Laurie Orr, Scott and Kathy Brandwein and Farley Neuman and Sheila Brown, for helping me feel at home, temporarily, in a faraway place during treatment in California. Across the country in New York, I owe humble thanks to Helene Rubinstein, David Granger, Peter Griffin, John Korpics and John Kenney, all at *Esquire*, where this book got its start. I also thank Katie Couric of NBC's *Today* for helping my story find more readers, and for showing me that private parts and public education do go hand in hand. Across the Atlantic, Chris Sulavik of Tatra Press and Jim Moscou offered key advice and editing suggestions at stops along England's Lane and Haverstock Hill. Michael Schrage, Allison Ryan, Bob Condor and Viki Psihoyos all helped to make this book as reader-friendly as it is personal. Eric Kampmann and Gail Kump at Midpoint Trade Books helped make it more than widely available. My gratitude goes to Flip Brophy and Cia Glover at Sterling Lord Literistic for their enduring friendship and guidance. And I owe thanks to all my dear friends in and around Boulder, Colorado, who pitched in and helped make our home feel just like that, instead of a hospital ward, between the tiresome chemotherapy "tours."

To my dear sons, Dad says, Thanks, guys for all the wisdom and joy you share each day. Finally, thank you, Paula, for teaching me what soul mate actually means. You gave me, along with more love and support than any partner has a right to ask for, no other option than to fight with everything I had, to become a survivor.

Epilog

On October 4, 2004, I drove more than 40 miles to Denver to see six-time Tour de France champion (and cancer survivor) Lance Armstrong ride less than one mile on his bike. I went mostly to show support of his maiden, cross-country "Tour of Hope" charity ride, designed to improve the lives of countless cancer patients, survivors and their families. But truth be told, I also attended to find out what it feels like to "join" the fraternity of survivors in person, instead of merely in print. At work sometimes, at neighborhood barbecues; to many people I don't know that well, I'm "that guy who had colon cancer." At the Armstrong event, I'd be just another cancer dude, one among hundreds. Under leaden skies, unusual for Colorado that time of year, I climbed a short hill to get a better view, and watched the motorcycle police escort—all serious-like, in formation with swirling-flashing cop lights—part the milling crowd of about 2,000 people as they led Lance and his entourage to a podium behind the University of Colorado's Health Sciences Cancer Center. It felt pretty comfortable; I certainly wasn't alone.

After a couple quick warm-up jokes (including an unscripted dig at our leaders for spending $200 billion on Iraq instead of on cancer research at home), Armstrong thanked the crowd, his doctors, his fellow riders and the millions who'd bought the dollar "Live Strong" bracelets his foundation has sold. He then thanked the Bristol-Myers Squibb company for making the chemotherapy drugs that helped save his life. Then he left, too soon it seemed. I wanted more; I wanted to feel the Armstrong "aura." Even though, I realized, after starting his Tour in California the week prior, he was only as far as the Rockies… and he had to pedal his self to Washington, D.C., with other survivor-cyclists, by next week. So I understood. I picked up my free energy bars, anti-cancer brochures and bottle of spring water and took off.

"On a bicycle, you never know what's around the next bend," Armstrong has said, "when a view may open up, or [when] the Alps may shear off into the sea."

Incredibly, less than 30 minutes later, driving home on Highway 470, I witnessed for the first time in my life, a tornado—not on TV, but out on the plains. My view had opened up alright: I saw a funnel cloud swirling slowly, hovering ominously, maybe 8 to 10 miles away. The tornado was east of the Rocky Mountains and populated areas, to be sure, but not far enough east for my comfort. Sightings had hit the radio airwaves, and a half-dozen, goofball storm chasers stopped their cars to "get video." Me, I hit the gas and, as Lance might say, tried to put it in my rearview in a hurry. On a bike, on a highway, in the gloom of an oncologist's office, turns out you never do know what's around the next bend.

In fact, I wrote this book to help survivors and their families navigate the territory "round the next bend"—whether that means four months till the next CT scan...or four years till cancer-free "cure." I also wrote this book because I believe every cancer patient can take a bit more control of his or her body, in a positive way. But don't take it from me: Listen to Dr. Barrie Cassileth, an expert in healing therapies at Memorial Sloan-Kettering Cancer Center, when she told me, in speaking of acupuncture: "We used to think the gains were due to a placebo effect. But that can't be said to be true for children and animal studies, and they have both shown positive effects." Pets, after all, simply have no way of "faking" feeling better. I wrote this book because the terrain of healing is changing as well, and most every survivor can use (at least parts of) a field guide of sorts.

As survivors and patients in the mid-2000s, we now know major advances have been made since 1995 in terms of curing and managing colorectal cancer. And while colon cancer may still lag behind breast and prostate cancer in the public consciousness and research dollars, it's gaining. And quickly. Where surgeons and doctors used to have just a few choices when it came to treating their patients for colorectal cancer, some now bemoan there are too many choices! In some ways the science has outstripped the practice of medicine. The proof is that docs admit they often aren't sure which drug to use first. But as doctors and patients (and their families) have told me or shown me time and again in these pages, there is more than a little reason to be optimistic. As I've come to learn, as an ex-patient who once was starving just to hear that I was, potentially, "curable," there is real reason to believe that in our lifetimes, colorectal cancer will lose and survivors will win.

ABOUT THE AUTHOR

Curtis Pesmen, author of *How a Man Ages*, *What She Wants* and *Your First Year of Marriage,* and who has written for *Esquire*, *GQ*, *SELF*, *Glamour*, *Redbook* and *Outside* magazines, was diagnosed with advanced colon cancer in 2001. As health/features editor of *SELF* magazine, he helped develop the internationally recognized, pink-ribbon breast cancer awareness campaign. An award-winning, seven-part series of Pesmen's (so far) successful fight against colon cancer was featured in *Esquire* magazine in 2001 and 2003. He lives in Boulder, Colorado, with his wife, Paula, film producer and founder of There With Care, and two young sons.

Contact: Curtis Pesmen
c/o STERLING LORD LITERISTIC, INC.
MS. FLIP BROPHY
65 BLEECKER ST.
NEW YORK, NY 10012
(212) 780-6050

www.bocomedia.com